T0107094

"By massaging acupoints on the scalp and face, one can treat the entire body. The Head is the capital of the human body and is the confluence of all the Yin & Yang Meridians."

—*The Yellow Emperor's Canon of Internal Medicine*
(First Book on Chinese Medicine)

DR.WU'S HEAD MASSAGE

DR. WU'S HEAD MASSAGE

ANTI-AGING AND HOLISTIC HEALING THERAPY

Dr. Bin Jiang Wu

YMAA Publication Center
Wolfeboro, NH USA

YMAA Publication Center, Inc.
Main Office
 PO Box 480
 Wolfeboro, NH, 03894
 1-800-669-8892 • www.ymaa.com • info@ymaa.com

© 2005 by Bin Jiang Wu

All rights reserved. No part of this book may be reproduced in any form, in either any form, either by Photostat, microfilm, xerography, or any other means, or incorporated in to any information retrieval system, electronic or mechanical, without the written permission of the copyright owner.

All rights reserved including the right of
reproduction in whole or in part in any form.

Editor: Susan Bullowa
Cover Design: Katya Popova
Anatomical figures and illustrations used by permission of Vincent Pratchett.
Organ and Body Parts Distribution Chart Copyright Dr. Bin Jiang Wu

ISBN-10: 1-59439-057-6
ISBN-13: 978-1-59439-057-9

20200513

Publisher's Cataloging in Publication

Wu, Bin Jiang.

Dr. Wu's head massage : anti-aging and holistic healing therapy /
Bin Jiang Wu. -- 1st ed. -- Boston, Mass. : YMAA Publication Center,
2005.

p. ; cm.

ISBN-13: 978-1-59439-057-9
ISBN-10: 1-59439-057-6
Includes bibliographical references and index.

1. Massage therapy. 2. Head--Massage. 3. Massage--China.
4. Medicine, Chinese. 5. Alternative medicine. I. Title.

RM723.C5 W8 2005   2005932449
615.8/22--dc22   0510

DISCLAIMER The information in this book is not meant as a substitute for medical treatment or advice. A person feeling ill should seek the consultation of his or her physician. This book is not written to replace your regular medical doctor or the medicine thereof, but for your knowledge and information. The author and the publisher are not responsible for any injury or illness that may occur as the result of following any of the instructions provided in this book.

Printed in USA.

Table of Contents

About Acupuncture Naming Conventions

The author uses The National Certification Commission for Acupuncture and Oriental Medicine (NCCAOM) standards for naming acupoints throughout this book.

Meridian	Name	Abbreviation
Hand Yangming	Large Intestine	LI
Foot Yangming	Stomach	ST
Hand Taiyang	Small Intestine	SI
Foot Taiyang	Urinary Bladder	UB
Hand Shaoyang	Triple Warmer/Sanjiao	SJ
Foot Shaoyang	Gall Bladder	GB
Du Mai	Governing Vessel	GV (Du)
Ren Mai	Conception Vessel	CV (Ren)

Dedication

This book is dedicated to my beloved parents and to those teachers whose guidance is indispensable to me.

Forward by Dr. Xue Tai Wan

Chinese medicinal massage, also called Tuina, has been around for a very long time. According to historical records, in the 7th century B.C. Bian Que, a renowned doctor in China integrated acupuncture, Tuina, and Chinese herbs to help save the dying Crown Prince. For over 2000 years since the Han Dynasty, *The Yellow Emperor's Canon of Internal Medicine* has established the principles of Chinese medicinal massage.

Chinese medicinal massage is a branch of Chinese medicine that is unlike western massage. The primary difference is that Chinese medicinal massage uses theories of channels and acupoints to achieve its goals. Massaging part of the body will enable the healing of the whole body. There is an emphasis on methods and techniques of manipulation that will not only relieve stress, but also fatigue. The ultimate purpose, however, is to enhance self-preservation and treat disease.

Head Massage is quite important in Chinese medicinal massage. According to Traditional Chinese Medicine, the head is the juncture of all six Yin and Yang Channels that are joined by two more significant channels the GV (Du) and CV (Ren). The brain becomes the ocean of marrow where all channels meet and are controlled and monitored. By massaging the head's acupoints, it stimulates Qi, and helps the circulation of Qi and blood. This improves the internal organs, and the body's functioning and overall health. According to western theory, the brain is the most sophisticated part of the body's nervous system. The central nervous system controls the brain, and activity is triggered in the brain cells. In head massage, this excitement is balanced through touch, thus improving not only the brain's circulation, but also the body's general health.

Dr. Wu earned his Masters Degree from the most prominent medical university in China—The China Academy of Traditional Chinese Medicine (Beijing). He specializes in acupuncture, Chinese medicinal massage, and Qigong. He has combined medical theory with his expertise and experience to develop a unique method of head massage focusing on the different head regions. Dr. Wu's innovations are significant not only to the Chinese medical profession, but to the general public as well. The publishing of this book will increase public awareness of this new development.

It is my privilege to recognize Dr. Wu's outstanding contribution to both medical knowledge and to our society.

—Dr. Xue Tai Wang March 24, 2000. Beijing, China
Dr. Xue Tai Wang is a world-renowned scientist
in the fields of acupuncture and is the Past President of
the World Federation of Acupuncture Moxibustion Society

Preface

When I graduated from high school in 1972, I was caught up in the Chinese Cultural Revolution. All the universities were closed and graduating students were sent out to the country for further "labor training." I went back to my small hometown village in Hebai province to learn Chinese medicine with my uncle. One day I had the flu and my head was in severe pain. One old Chinese doctor in the medical clinic performed about 10 minutes of head massage on me, and immediately my headache was relieved. Right then I became an apprentice under the old doctor to study this massage form. His great-grandfather was an imperial doctor during the late Qing dynasty, and this head massage was handed down from the Imperial Palace. It was said that the Empress Dowager Chi Xi was especially fond of one eunuch named Small An because he would massage her, particularly on the head before she rose every morning.

In 1977 when the Cultural Revolution ended and University entrance resumed, I entered Heilongjiang TCM University and obtained my Bachelor of Medicine. In 1985, I entered the China Academy of Traditional Chinese Medicine in Beijing and obtained my Masters of Medicine (Qigong) in 1988. It was the first session of a Masters Degree of Medicine Qigong program in China and the world. During my studies in the university and the academy, I developed my fundamental theories based on the many ancient head massage literature I had looked up. Also included in the head massage techniques are many different folk therapies: Shaolin, Er-Mei, Qigong, and other Tuina techniques.

WHM is rooted in Traditional Chinese Medicine's basic theories of Yin/Yang, Five Elements, and the Meridian System. The basis of TCM is to activate and supplement the body's innate healing capacity to restore biological balance and harmony.

All medicine arises out of the need to avoid pain and keep illness and disability at bay, and to lead a healthy and full life.

With the progress of technology and widespread use of computers, we have seen an increasing number of people confined to the office. These so-called "office groups" constitute a large part of modern society. Computer programmers, secretaries, managers, accountants, doctors, lawyers, are just some of the typical white-collar professionals. Ironically, these "office groups" come to be the most susceptible victims of modern civilization.

For instance, the fast-paced stressful city life is related to irregularities of bowel movement, insomnia, and many more disorders. Instead of walking, we now use driving as a means of transportation. At work, we sit in front of the computer, and at home, we sit in front of the TV. Yes, modern inventions serve us well, but at the same time, a train of civilization-related illnesses, such as vertigo, irritability, headache, visual fatigue, heavy shoulders, and insomnia, flares up alongside the computer, the car, and the Internet.

The decreased physical exertion and increased neck, eye and brain activities reflect the dramatic revolution of the modern society from, say, a hundred years ago. A challenging question confronts us in the face of the rapidly changing society: Is there a natural approach to address the illnesses that are rooted in the modern civilization? The development of the Wu's Head Massage is the response to the call of the above problems.

Regardless of whether it is traditional or modern, massages in the world have never been focused on the head and the face. While there have been few manipulations and acupoints applied on the scalp and facial area, the emphasis was nonetheless on the body trunk and the four limbs. The omission of head massage is probably tied to the fact that throughout history, physical labor had always been the predominant (if not the only) force in the labor market. Nevertheless, the constitution of the modern labor market is no longer the same since the progress of technology has transformed the way we live. Instead of heavy physical work, the white-collar workers now require vigorous mental work. Moreover, all these dramatic shifts took place only within the past fifty years or so.

Needless to say, the head and neck are important parts of the body. TCM states:

> "Head is the residence of the consciousness and the mind. If the head is tilted, the vision is impaired and the consciousness is exhausted. The head is the capital of the human body and it is the confluence of all the Yin and Yang meridians."

Both meridians and acupoints are rather dense in the area of the head and the face. The meridians and collaterals are the pathways in which the Qi and blood of the human body are circulated, forming a network and linking the head/face and the body/limb into an organic whole.

Therefore, certain zones of the head/face could reflect the dynamic states of diseases. By massaging these areas to promote the Qi and blood flow in the related meridians, balancing the Yin and Yang energy—not only the problem of the head/face—but also the relevant organ/limb can be treated. Moreover, as a bonus, it has the cosmetic effect of resisting the aging process.

The theoretical basis of Wu's Head Massage is found in the *Yellow Emperor's Canon of Internal Medicine*. It is said in the Chapter of Miraculous Pivot, "different zones of the face pertain to different body/limbs." To facilitate study and practice, we have devised a pictorial distribution of organs/limbs on the face as described in the *Yellow Emperor's Canon of Internal Medicine*. (See Figure 6-1)

In addition to the foundation of the experiences of our ancestors, we have assimilated the theories of the head and auricular acupunctures, Shaolin and Er-Mei acupoint pressure techniques, Qigong, and hypnosis.

Extensive clinical and teaching experiences in Asia, Europe, and North America have provided the basis of further refinement, thereby establishing the complete set of guidance to both the theoretical and practical levels of the Wu's Head Massage. This complete set of meridian-based head massage techniques fulfills the mission of massaging an essential area that was once neglected.

Wu's Head Massage directly stimulates the head, and the face and neck regions, resulting in a sedative and lulling effect, and balancing the Yin and Yang energy. Thus, it achieves excellent therapeutic results for diseases of modern civilization that are manifested on the head and neck, as well as improving the aesthetic appearance, and prolonging our life span.

The points and areas stimulated during Wu's Head Massage have been used by acupuncturists for a wide range of applications. Many diseases have been treated successfully. These include diseases in the nervous, respiratory, motor, cardiovascular, gastrointestinal, urinary, five-senses, and gynecological systems. Among the most noteworthy is sequela resulting from various forms of cerebral cranium damage like cerebral hemorrhage, meningitis, and cerebral embolism.

More than ten years have passed since the presentation of Wu's Head Massage in 1993 in an article at the Third World Acupuncture and Moxibustion Conference in Japan. Clinical observation in Asia, Europe, and North America has proved that the method is easy to learn, yet fast acting with no side effects. It is necessary, however, that each individual understands that the ultimate responsibility for our health lies upon each of us as individuals.

To increase the benefits of WHM and Chinese medicine in general, we must take control of our diets, sleep habits, work styles, and exercise. All of these will inevitably influence how successful we will be at re-establishing harmony within our bodies, our lives, and nature. The principles of WHM do not have to await the arrival of illness. Prevention is the key according to Chinese medicine.

This authoritative guide to Chinese massage for the head and neck will provide its readers with a deep understanding of this extraordinary and ancient system of healing.

Acknowledgements

Special thanks in writing this book, I have received much advice and guidance from many individuals. I would like to express my sincere gratitude and thanks to Dr. Xue Tai Wang, Professor Jin Zhang, and Dr. Adam Chen for their theoretical advice. I also give thanks to Ming Xia, Qi Wen Li, Hong Yu, James Huang, Mona Bolton, John Li, and Vincent Pratchett who have helped me greatly in the research, typing and graphic design of this book. Thanks to Maggie Cheung and Pei-Ling Chang for their proofreading efforts. Class and park photos by Robert Liew and Robert Lowe. Special thanks to my wife, Dr. Yi Ling Zhang, for her continual support and in the area of research and her behind the scene efforts. Without the contributions of all these people, this book would not be possible.

Dr. Bin Jiang Wu
The Ontario College of Traditional Chinese Medicine
145 Sheppard Ave. E. Suite 201
Toronto, Ontario
Canada M2N 3A7
Tel: 416-222-3667
Fax: 416-646-3667

Mission Statement

My mission is to present and teach Wu's Head-Massage to the world.

Preparing a mission statement is a serious task because stating the objective also provides the standard with which to judge success or failure. Serious however does not mean complicated, it means honest. From honesty comes simplicity and from this quiet simplicity springs clarity. I am a doctor and a teacher, so my life's work revolves around healing and educating. Who? Anyone with a serious interest that takes the time and trouble to knock on my door.

A doctor's primary mission is health, but the western and oriental concept of promoting health differs greatly. In the West, a doctor that cures a terrible disease is a great doctor, but in China, the best doctor is the one who's patient did not get sick at all! Becoming a Western doctor or a doctor of Traditional Chinese Medicine (TCM) does have at least one common characteristic though. Both require many years of discipline and study.

Wu's Head Massage (WHM) was created by using my knowledge of TCM to consult and research the Chinese classical medical texts. Chinese medicine with its long history and unique terminology is not an easy study. What began many years ago as an academic and scholarly endeavor has been refined by clinical study, and has yielded a profound yet easy to learn anti-aging and holistic healing therapy. The complete WHM sequence is composed of sixty parts, called movements.

Although learning medicine is a difficult process, learning health and how to heal is not. When children get hurt they rub and cradle the injured area. As the tears flow, they wipe them away and hold their head in their hands. The parent will often fix the problem with a kiss and a soothing hug. Therefore, from the earliest stages in life healing can be looked upon as something personal, natural, and simple. It begins with a touch.

The importance of the head in relation to healing and health cannot be overstated. It occupies the highest central position of the body, and it is the residence of mental, spiritual, and physical characteristics unique to every individual. Ironically, Wu's Head Massage is not about massaging the head. More accurately, it is about improving the health of the whole body by using the head as the key.

The purpose and intent of this book is two-fold. First, it will outline the principles theory and science behind the therapy thus serving as a reference source. More importantly however, it will provide the reader with a practical hands-on guide for learning and applying Wu's Head massage. Armed with a sincere interest in TCM or massage, the reader can begin self or social practice of this complete holistic health therapy almost immediately. Professional certification at our school requires 60 hours of class and clinical study.

The most important characteristic of a health practitioner is not how much they know, but how well they touch. Doing the illustrated WHM sequence as correctly as possible will naturally lead to a deeper understanding of its underlying principles over time.

In TCM theory, energy never really ends. It transforms into something else, so that an end is often really only a beginning. From the moment the reader begins to perform the WHM sequence, my mission reaches completion. Education through touch leading simply to practicing health. It is hoped that at the point where my mission finds completion, the reader's mission may be just beginning. Health begins with a simple touch.

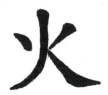

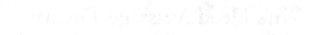

Chapter 1

The Foundation of Traditional Chinese Medicine

To understand what WHM is all about, it is important to have at least a basic understanding of Traditional Chinese Medicine (TCM).

Chinese medicine is a system of healing that has evolved over the last 3,000 years and is based on a profound philosophy and a rich empirical tradition. It has produced a highly sophisticated set of practices designed to cure illness and to maintain health and well-being. These practices include acupuncture, herbal medicine, massage, diet, moving and static exercise (Qigong, Taiji, and internal exercises).

The *Huang Di Nei Jing* (*The Yellow Emperor's Canon of Internal Medicine*) dating to the third century B.C. also contained much older material and was one of the first written accounts of the various theories of TCM, including the theories of Yin/Yang and the Five Elements. This ancient text is one of the earliest accounts of the effectiveness of massaging the head to treat the whole body.

Yin/Yang & Five Elements Theory

The theories of Yin/Yang and the Five Elements originated in ancient China, and form the perspectives and methodologies applied to understand nature. Yin/Yang and the Five Element Theory constitute an ancient Chinese cosmology to explain nature, as well as materialism and dialectics in ancient China.

These two theories have exerted a great deal of influence on the development of various kinds of science in ancient China, such as astronomy, meteorology, calendar, agronomy, biology, chemistry, medicine, and so on. They were even assimilated by specific subjects, and became the theoretical basis of academic development. TCM is one of these subjects. Medical experts in ancient China applied the two theories mainly to explain the entire relationship between a human body and nature, the organization, physiological functions and pathological changes in the body, and to guide diagnosis and treatment.

Yin/Yang

The ancients held that the material world was generated and developed in the opposite movement between Yin-Qi and Yang-Qi. Yin and Yang represent not only the two opposite material forces in the natural world, but also the two aspects of contradiction. This ancient concept holds that the material world is constantly generating, developing, and changing due to the interaction of Yin and Yang.

Seeing that everything can be divided into two aspects, the Yin/Yang concept was applied to explain duality and delineates that by opposition and support and sometimes synthesis; the ebb and flow of Yin and Yang is intrinsic in everything.

The Yin/Yang theory holds that the world is a whole, the result of the unity of opposites, Yin and Yang. The motion of the opposites is responsible for change in the universe. Ying and Yang represent properties that oppose and interconnect. Rapid, outward, ascending movement, warmth, heat, and brightness pertain to Yang. Stillness and inward, descending movement, coldness and dullness belong to Yin. When speaking of Yin and Yang in the medical field, functions possessing promoting, warming and exciting actions, and so on all belong to Yang, while those responsible for condensing, moistening and restraining actions, and so on belong to Yin.

The properties of Yin and Yang are by no means absolute, but relative. Relativity is maintained by transformation of Yin and Yang. It is manifested in the unlimited division of everything. For instance, daytime is Yang and night is Yin.

When treating an illness or disease in Chinese medicine, we consider the root cause as the disharmony between Yin and Yang, the basic therapeutic principle is to regain a balance between Yin and Yang by regulating them through reinforcing the deficient one and reducing the excess. The Yin/Yang theory guides the treatment and is used to determine the therapeutic principle and to summarize properties of drugs.

Five Elements Theory

Like the Yin/Yang Theory, the Five Elements Theory has become a part of the TCM system of medicine. The Five Elements Theory holds that wood, fire, earth, metal and water are the most basic and essential substances. Their movement and change constitute the material world. The Five Elements Theory expounds that everything is formed by the motion and change of these five basic substances and the relationships of mutual generation and mutual restraint exist among these five elements. Nothing is isolated and motionless, but everything keeps a kinetic balance in the incessant movement of these elements. The theory of the five elements is used to explore the constitutional form of all things, and the way in which they move and change.

The characteristics of wood apply to all things that have an action or feature of flourishing growth corresponding to wood. All things characterized by warmth, heat, and ascending action correspond to fire. All things that have generating, transmuting, carrying, and receiving actions correspond to earth. All things that have clearing, descending, and astringent actions correspond to metal. All things that are cold and cool, moist, and moving downward correspond to water.

Each of the main 12 organs in the body, both the six Yin (zang organs): heart, pericardium, liver, kidneys, lungs, and spleen and the six Yang (fu organs): stomach, large intestine, small intestine, bladder, gall bladder, and Sanjiao, can be characterized by a particular element.

Vital Substances

In TCM, we commonly refer to and work with a number of vital substances found within the body. What follows is a brief description of these substances.

Qi

Qi is the vital principle that continuously moves in the body. Body fluids is a general term for normal aqueous liquids within the body. When classified according to their respective properties into Yin and Yang, Qi has promoting and warming actions, pertaining to Yang, while blood and body fluids are liquid, nourishing and moistening, and pertain to Yin.

The energy that tissues and organs, such the viscera (12 organs) and meridians, need for their physiological activities originate from Qi, blood, and body fluids. Metabolism depends upon the normal physiological functions of the tissues and organs, such as the viscera and meridians. Therefore, a close relationship exists between the tissues and organs in physiopathology. Moreover, there is also the basic matter consisting of the body.

The Qi of the body originates from three forms: from prenatal jing (Vital Principle), inherited from parents, nutrients from food, and clear Qi (air). Qi is formed by combining the three through the functions of internal organs.

Prenatal jing can be fully effective only by depending upon the function of jing in the kidney; refined nutrients in water and cereals (diet) can be ingested and derived from food only with the help of the transporting and digesting functions of the spleen and stomach. Clear Qi (air) can be inspired by depending on the lung. Qi is formed by the physiological functions of the kidneys, spleen, stomach and lung. Only if the physiological functions of the kidneys, spleen and stomach, lung, and other organs are normal and harmonious, can Qi be properly created. If these functions fail to remain normal, pathological changes occur, such as deficient Qi, etc.

For the formation of Qi, the transporting and digesting function of the spleen and stomach are important. This is because after birth, the body depends upon food to maintain its activities. The body's capacity to ingest nutrients from food depends upon the receiving, transporting, and digesting functions of the spleen and stomach, so that food can be digested and absorbed. Jing is dependent upon the nutrients in food.

Qi is classified by a number of different names according to its component location and functions.

Primordial Qi

Derived from jing, stored in the kidneys. Whether it flourishes or not depends on prenatal endowment and is related to gastrosplenic functions of the transporting and digesting refined matter from food. It flows through the body via the Triple Warmer (Sanjiao). Its main task is to promote the growth and development of the body, and to warm and stimulate various tissues and organs.

Chest Qi

Stored in the thorax. It is composed of a combination of Clear Qi (air) absorbed by the lung and refined matter from food transported and digested by the spleen and stomach. It promotes respiration by passing through the respiratory tract, and promotes Qi and blood circulation by pouring Qi into the Heart Meridian.

Nutritional Qi

Flows within the meridians together with blood. It pertains to Yin. It originates from food and is derived from the essential part of the refined food. It nourishes the body and generates blood.

Defensive Qi

This Qi flows outside the meridians. It is Yang and is derived from the refined principle of food. It is strong, active and moves rapidly. It protects the body surface and prevents the invasion of exogenous pathogenic factors by nourishing the viscera, muscles, skin and hair, and other organs, regulating and controlling the opening and closing of the junction between the skin and muscle, and excreting sweat so as to keep a relatively stable body temperature.

Blood

Blood is one of the fundamental substances that constitute the body. By circulating within the vessels, blood brings nutrition to the cells. Blood is chiefly composed of Nutritional Qi and body fluids. Since the nutritional principle and body fluids originate from the refined matter from food that has been digested and absorbed by the spleen and stomach, the spleen and stomach are the source of Qi and blood. Blood can be generated through the actions of Nutritional Qi and the lung.

As a whole, Nutritional Qi and body fluids are the main basis for the formation of blood. Since both Nutritional Qi and body fluids originate from the refined matter from food, whether dietary nutrients are rich or not and whether the transporting and digesting functions of the spleen and stomach are strong or not, directly influence the formation of blood. A prolonged insufficiency of nutrients or prolonged disharmony of the transporting and digesting functions of the spleen and stomach may lead to insufficient blood.

In addition, there is a relationship between jing and blood. Jing is stored in the kidney and blood is stored in the liver. If the vital principle in the kidney is full, the liver will be well nourished, and blood enriched; if the liver stores enough blood, the kidney will have enough vital principle. Hence, "jing and blood originate from the same source."

Blood nourishes and moistens the entire body. It circulates in the vessels and reaches the viscera and skin, muscles, tendons and bones and continuously nourishes and moistens the viscera, tissues, and organs to keep physiological activities at a normal level.

Blood is Yin in nature and is concerned with calmness. Normal blood circulation is determined by the harmony or balance between the promoting and controlling actions of Qi.

Body Fluids

Body fluids include fluids within the various viscera, tissues and organs, and normal secretions (e.g., gastric fluid, intestinal fluid, nasal discharge, tears). Body fluids are fundamental to life.

Jin (clear and thin fluid) and ye (turbid and thick fluid) are the two main body fluids originating from diet and dependent upon the transporting and digesting functions of the spleen and stomach. Body fluids originate from diet. They are formed in the stomach from the refined matter from food and the small intestine differentiating the purified nutrients from the turbid material and upwardly transporting the nutrients to the spleen. They are distributed and excreted chiefly through the transportation of the spleen and by the spreading and descending actions of the lung and the kidney, and the distributing function of the Triple Warmer.

Body fluids are moistening and nourishing. Those distributed over the body surface moisten the hair and muscles; those pouring into the sense organs moisten and protect the eyes, nose, mouth, and other organs; those permeating blood have the action of nourishing and smoothing blood; those pouring into tissues and organs nourish and moisten the tissues and organs of various viscera; those exuding into bones nourish and moisten the marrow, spinal cord and brain.

The Meridians

The Meridian Theory includes the physiological functions, pathological changes, and interrelationships of the viscera. The meridians are the pathways in which the Qi and blood circulate in the body through which the viscera and limbs are connected. Most of the meridians (jing) run in the deep portion of the body, while their collaterals (luo) are in the superficial part of the body, some of which are exposed on the body surface.

Twelve Regular Meridians

The meridians are divided into regular and extraordinary meridians. There are 12 regular meridians that are divided into 3 pairs of Yin meridians and three pairs of Yang meridians on the hands and feet. These are the main passages in which Qi and blood circulate. Each of the twelve meridians connects with one of the 12 organs (viscera). The eight extraordinary meridians regulate the 12 regular meridians.

The Meridian Theory holds that the musculofascia meridians are a system, where Qi stagnates, gathers, scatters, and links with tendons, fascia, muscles and joints as well as the affiliated part of the twelve meridians, hence called the musculofascia meridians. They connect the four extremities and various tissues and control the activities of the twelve meridians on the body surface and where meridian Qi is distributed. The skin is divided into 12 parts corresponding to the 12 meridians, called the "twelve cutaneous areas of meridians."

The 12 meridians are symmetrically distributed over both sides of the body, and run respectively through the medial or lateral side of the upper or lower limb. Each meridian respectively pertains to a zang (Yin) or fu (Yang) organ. So, each of the 12 meridian names must include either hand/foot, Yin/Yang viscera.

Eight Extraordinary Meridians

The eight extraordinary meridians is a general term for the Governor Vessel Meridian, Conception Vessel Meridian, Strategic Vessel Meridian, Girdle Vessel Meridian, Mobility Vessel Meridian of Yin, Mobility Vessel Meridian of Yang, and the Regulating Vessel Meridian of Yin, Regulating Vessel Meridian of Yang. They are so called because they are not distributed as regularly as the 12 meridians; they are not directly connected with the viscera, and they differ from the twelve meridians.

These meridians strengthen the connection of the 12 meridians, and combines all the Yang and Yin meridians, controls all meridians, connects meridians in lumbar and abdominal regions, un-obstructs the upper and lower parts of the body, and irrigates the three Yin meridians and three Yang meridians. They also regulate Qi and blood in the 12 meridians.

Summary

In summary, to learn and apply Wu's Head Massage requires the practitioner to have a general understanding of the philosophy and foundation of TCM and a working knowledge of the body's energetic system.

The Earth has rivers and ocean currents and we use meridian lines to chart and navigate them. The Chinese view human beings in a similar way.

The body has channels through which health-giving energy (Qi) flows. These too are called meridians, and are named after the internal organ with which they share a special relationship. There are 12 regular meridians that branch cross and interact. Where they flow along the surface, they can be influenced and manipulated at concavities and points. These numbered points are called acupoints. Energy flows from the lowest to the highest number.

The Chinese divide the body into Yin and Yang. Yang (active) can be thought of as where the sunshine would hit directly. Likewise, Yin (passive) would be the areas the sun does not reach directly. Therefore, meridians are Yin or Yang as well as upper and lower. If a person is standing with their arms up, the direction energy flows within the Yin meridians is up and Yang meridians down.

Unlike rivers that are usually separate, the body's energy rivers flow from one to the next in a continuous and orderly fashion. In a 24-hour time period, energy will have traveled through all the meridians and circulated the body three times. During this daily period, each meridian will have a 2-hour span of maximum and minimum influence.

In addition to the 12 regular meridians, there are two extraordinary ones that the Wu's Head Massage practitioner deals with. They are called Ren (Conception Vessel) and Du (Governing Vessel). These differ from the regular channels because they do not precede or succeed each other. They both start at the perineum and rise up front and back, ending their cycle by flowing through each other. (See Figure 1-1)

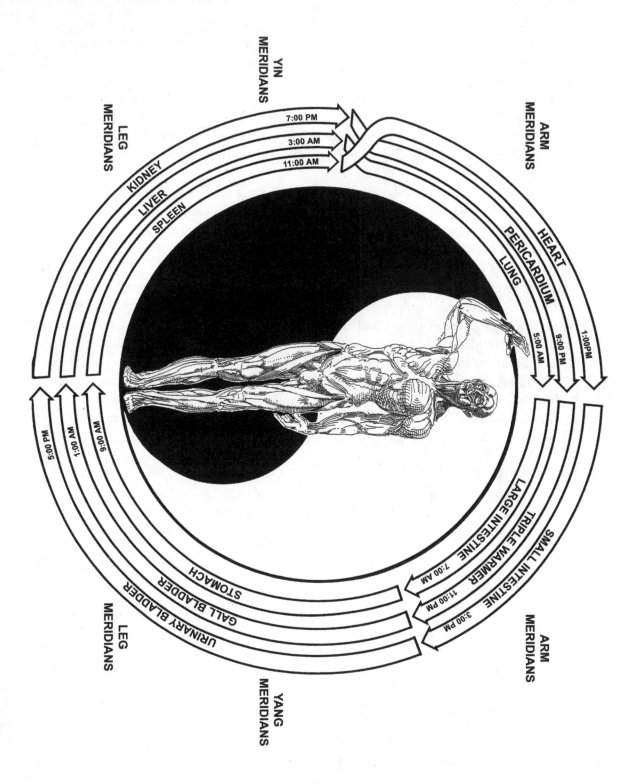

FIGURE 1-1 ARM AND LEG MERIDIANS

CHAPTER 2
Meridian Pathways of the Head, Face, and Neck

We will now have a look at the paths of the meridians, emphasizing the points that are directly related to the head face and neck (following pages).

The Path of the Large Intestine Meridian of the Hand—Yangming

1. The Large Intestine Meridian of Hand—Yangming begins at the tip of the index finger (Shangyang, LI 1).

2. Then travels to the highest point of the shoulder (Jianyu, LI 15).

3. Then along the anterior border of the acromion.

4. Up to the 7th cervical vertebrae (in Chinese Medicine, this point is extremely important because it is considered the confluence point of the three yang meridians of the hand and foot) (Dazhui (GV (Du) 14).

5. Then descends to Quepen (ST 12) the supraclavicular fossa.

6. One branch starts from Quepen (ST 12) and runs upward to the neck.

7. Then passes through the cheek.

8. And enters the lower gums.

9. Then it turns back to the upper lip and crosses the opposite meridian at the philtrum. From this point, the left meridian crosses to the right side of the face and the right meridian crosses over to the left side of the face to the edge of the nostrils (Yingxiang, LI 20). At this point the Large Intestine Meridian links with the Stomach Meridian of Foot—Yangming.

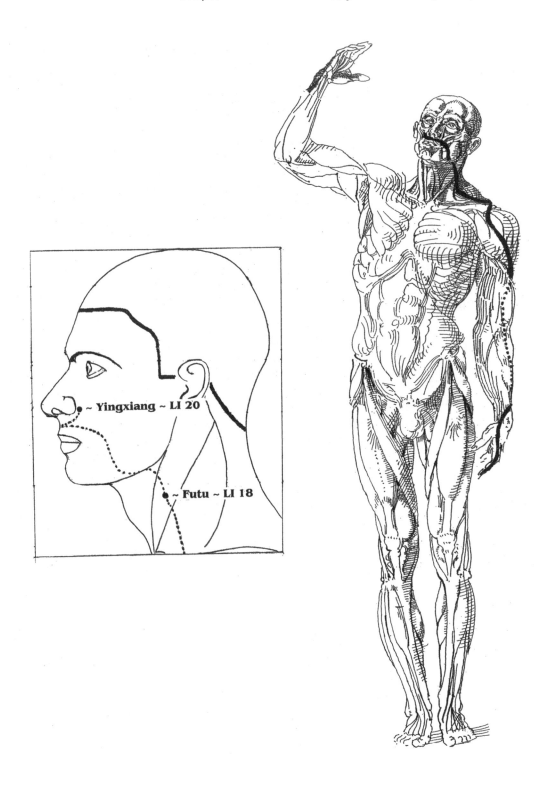

Figure 2-1 The Path of the Large Intestine Meridian of the Hand—Yangming

The Path of the Stomach Meridian of the Foot—Yangming

1. The Stomach Meridian of Foot—Yangming begins on the lateral side of the nasal ala.
2. Then ascends to the bridge of the nose, where it meets the Bladder Meridian of Foot—Taiyang.
3. Turning downwards along the lateral side of the nose.
4. It enters the upper gum.
5. Reemerging, it curves round the lips.
6. Then descends to meet the Ren Meridian at the mentolabial groove—Chengjiang (CV (Ren) 24).
7. It then runs posterolaterally across the lower portion of the cheek at Daying (ST 5).
8. Winding along the angle of the mandible—Jiache (ST 6).
9. It then ascends in front of the ear and traverses Shangguan (GB 3) of the Gallbladder, lips and Meridian of Foot—Shaoyang.
10. Then it follows the anterior hairline.
11. Until it reaches the forehead.
12. The facial branch emerging in front of Daying (ST 5) runs downwards to Renying (ST 9) From there it goes along the throat.
13. Then enters the supraclavicular fossa.
14. The pedal branch rises from the dorsum of the foot Chongyang (ST 42) and terminates at the medial side of the tip of the big toe, where it links with the Spleen Meridian of Foot—Taiyin.

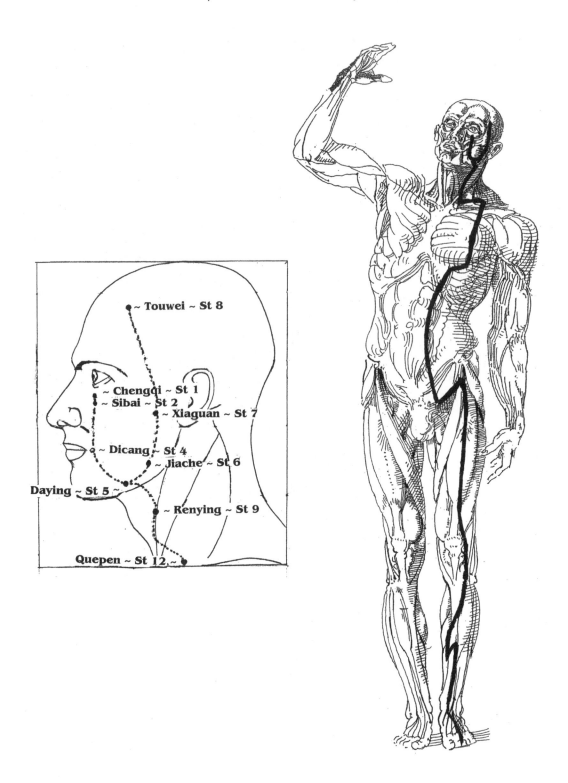

~ Touwei ~ St 8

~ Chengqi ~ St 1
~ Sibai ~ St 2
~ Xiaguan ~ St 7

~ Dicang ~ St 4
~ Jiache ~ St 6

Daying ~ St 5 ~

~ Renying ~ St 9

Quepen ~ St 12 ~

FIGURE 2-2 THE PATH OF THE STOMACH MERIDIAN OF FOOT—YANGMING

The Path of the Small Intestine Meridian of the Hand—Taiyang

1. The Small Intestine Meridian of Hand—Taiyang starts from the ulnar side of the tip of the little finger.
2. And continues up to the shoulder joint.
3. Then circles around the scapular region.
4. Till it meets Dazhui (GV (Du) 14) on the superior aspect of the shoulder.
5. Then, turns downwards to the supraclavicular fossa.
6. The branch from the supraclavicular fossa ascends along the neck.
7. To the cheek.
8. To the outer canthus.
9. And enters the ear.
10. The branch from the cheek runs upwards to the infraorbital region and further to the lateral side of the nose. Then it reaches the inner canthus to link with the Bladder Meridian of Foot—Taiyang.

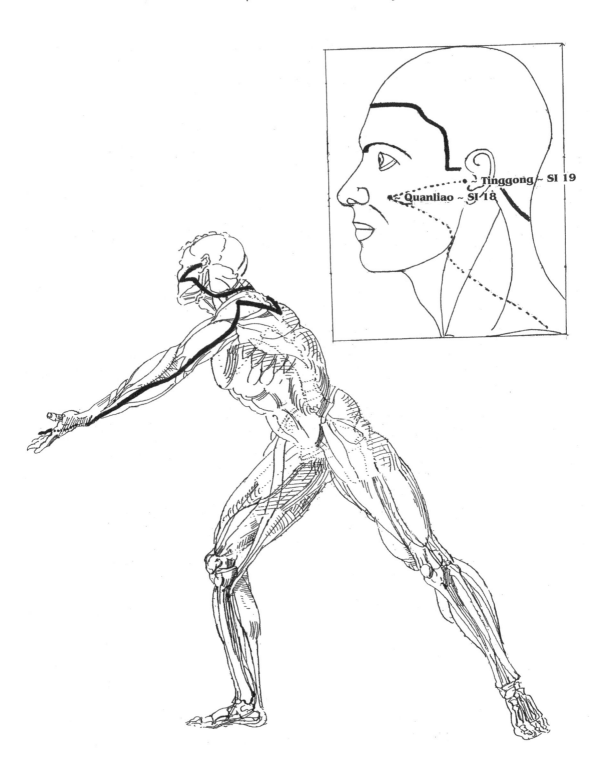

Tinggong ~ SI 19

Quanliao ~ SI 18

The Path of the Bladder Meridian of the Foot—Taiyang

1. The Bladder Meridian of Foot—Taiyang begins at the inner canthus.
2. Ascends to the forehead.
3. Then joins the Du Meridian at the vertex.
4. From the vertex, one branch arises and runs upwards to the temple.
5. The straight portion of the meridian enters and communicates with the brain from the vertex.
6. It then emerges and bifurcates. One branch descends along the nape of the neck.
7. Running downward along the medial aspect of the scapula region and parallel to the vertebral column.
8. The other branch runs straight downward along the medial border of the scapula.
9. And it reaches the lateral side of the tip of the little toe, and links with the Kidney Meridian of Foot—Shanyin.

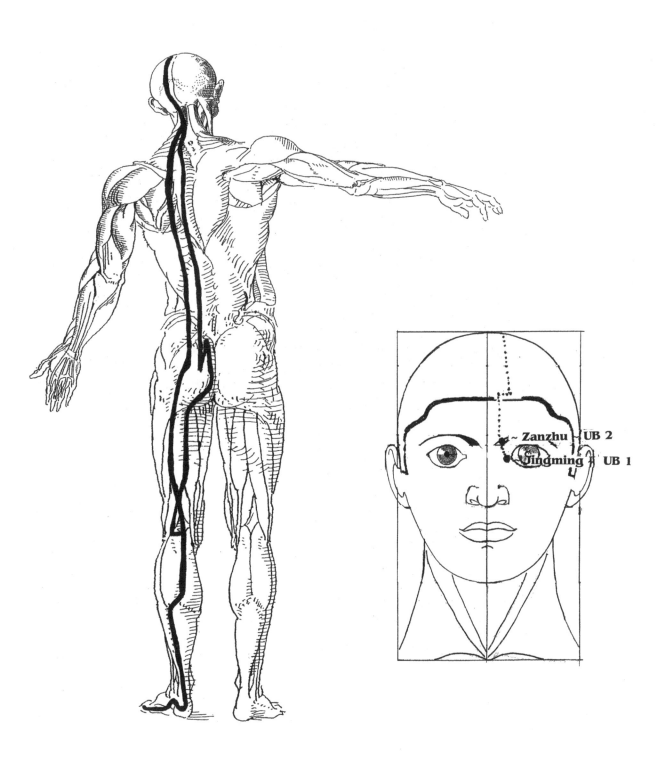

Zanzhu ─ UB 2

Jingming ─ UB 1

FIGURE 2-4 THE PATH OF THE BLADDER MERIDIAN OF FOOT—TAIYANG   19

The Path of the Sanjiao (Triple Warmer) Meridian of the Hand—Shaoyang

1. The Sanjiao Meridian of Hand—Shaoyang originates at the tip of the ring finger (Guanchong, SJ 1).
2. Then travels upwards along the arm until it reaches the shoulder region.
3. Where it crosses and passes behind the Gallbladder Meridian of Foot—Shaoyang.
4. It then winds over to the supraclaviculas fossa.
5. A branch rises from the chest and runs upwards.
6. And then emerges from the supraclavicular fossa.
7. From there, it ascends to the neck.
8. And runs along the posterior border of the ear.
9. And continues further to the corner of the anterior hairline.
10. From here it runs downwards to the cheek and terminates in the infraorbital region.
11. The auricular branch rises from the retroauricular region and enters the ear. Then it emerges in front of the ear, crosses the previous branch at the cheek.
12. And reaches the outer canthus to link with the Gallbladder Meridian of Foot—Shaoyang.

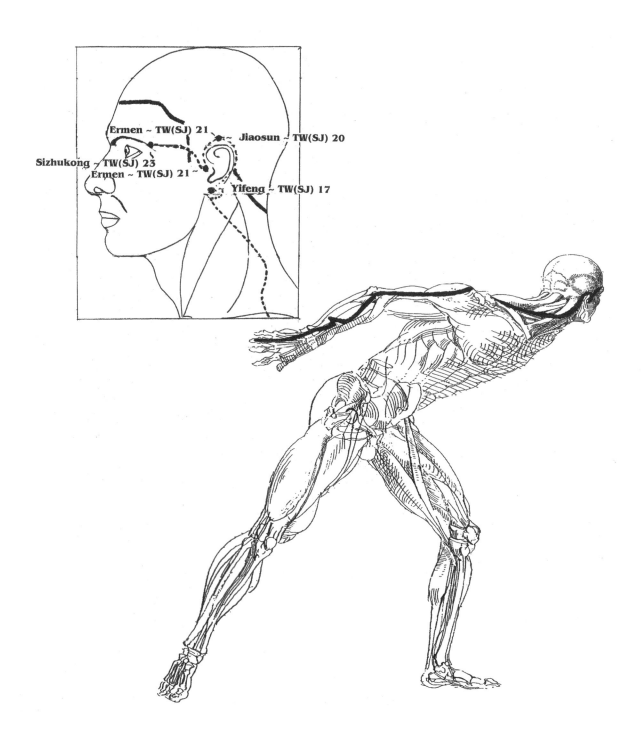

FIGURE 2-5 THE PATH OF THE SANJIAO (TRIPLE WARMER) MERIDIAN OF HAND—SHAOYANG   21

The Path of the Gallbladder Meridian of the Foot—Shaoyang

1. The Gallbladder Meridian of Foot—Shaoyang originates at the outer canthus (Tongziliao, GB 1).

2. Ascends to the corner of the forehead (Hanyan, GB 4).

3. Then curves downwards to the retroauricular region (Fengchi, GB 20).

4. And runs along the side of the neck in front of the Sanjiao Meridian of Hand—Shaoyang.

5. Down to the supraclavicular fossa.

6. The retroauricular branch rises from the retroauricular region and enters into the ear.

7. As it comes out of the ear it passes the preauricular region.

8. To the posterior aspect of the outer canthus.

9. The branch arising from the outer canthus

10. Runs downwards to Daying (ST 5).

11. And meets the Sanjiao Meridian of Hand—Shaoyang in the infraorbital region.

12. It then passes through Jiache (ST 6)

13. And descends to the neck, and enters the supraclavicular fossa where it meets the other branch which is already in the place. Here is where it links with the Liver Meridian of Foot—Jueyin.

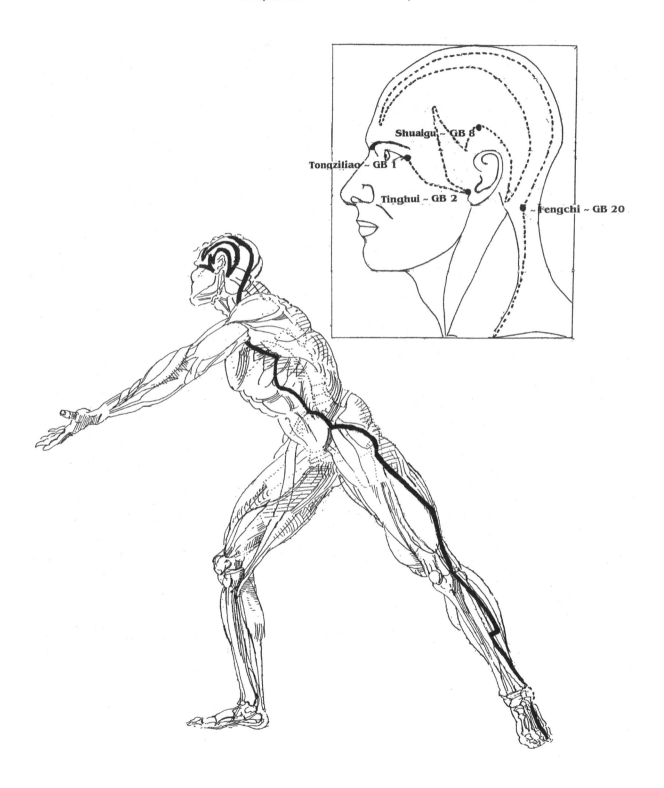

Shuaigu ~ GB 8

Tongziliao ~ GB 1

Tinghui ~ GB 2

~ Fengchi ~ GB 20

FIGURE 2-6 THE PATH OF THE GALLBLADDER MERIDIAN OF FOOT—SHAOYANG

The Path of the Du Meridian (Governing Vessel)

1. The Du Meridian arises from the lower abdomen and emerges from the perineum.

2. To Fengfu (GV (Du) 16) at the nape, where it enters the brain.

3. It further ascends to the vertex and winds along the forehead down to the nasal column.

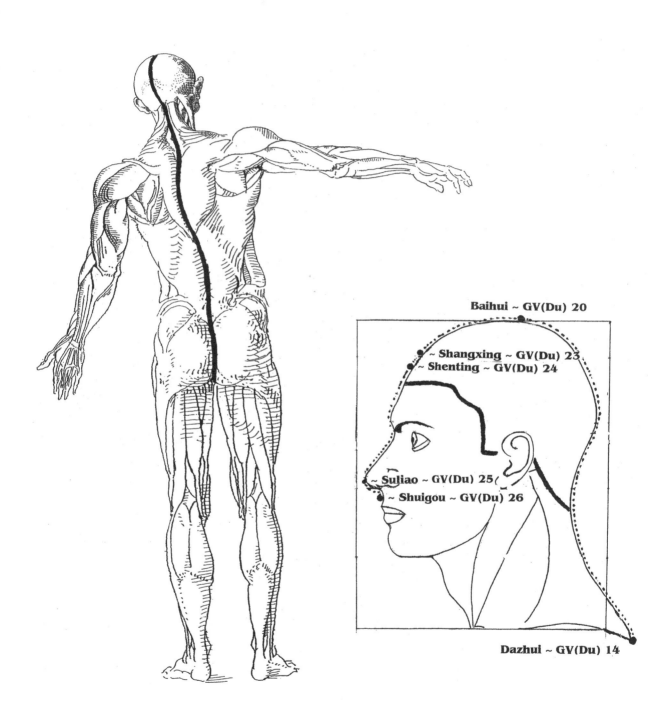

Baihui ~ GV(Du) 20

~ Shangxing ~ GV(Du) 23
~ Shenting ~ GV(Du) 24

~ Suliao ~ GV(Du) 25
~ Shuigou ~ GV(Du) 26

Dazhui ~ GV(Du) 14

FIGURE 2-7 THE PATH OF THE DU MERIDIAN

The Path of the Ren Meridian (Conception Vessel)

1. The Ren Meridian begins on the inside of the lower abdomen and emerges from the perineum.

2. And runs along the middle of the body toward the throat.

3. Ascending further, it curves around the lips.

4. Then passes through the cheek.

5. Then enters the infraorbital region.

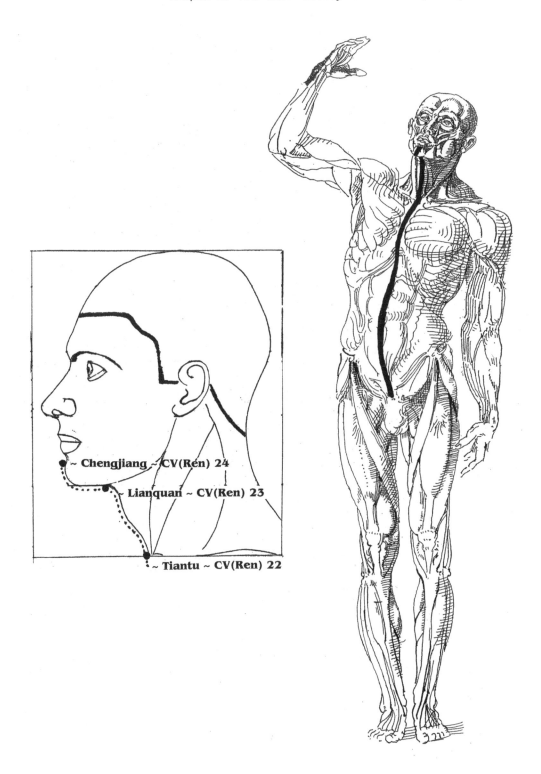

~ Chengjiang ~ CV(Ren) 24

Lianquan ~ CV(Ren) 23

~ Tiantu ~ CV(Ren) 22

FIGURE 2-8 THE PATH OF THE REN MERIDIAN 27

Part II
Acupoints on the Head

CHAPTER 3

Methods of Locating Acupoints

There are three commonly used methods that practitioners of TCM use to help them to accurately locate acupoints:
- Finger Measurement.
- Bone Proportional Measurement.
- Surface Anatomical Landmarks.

It is recommended that these methods be combined with one another when attempting to locate points, in order to guarantee more accuracy. The third method, Surface Anatomical Landmarks is, however, the most fundamental method while the other two are considered as supplemental methods.

Finger Measurement

For this method of locating acupoints, we use either the length or width of the patient's finger(s) as a measuring tool.

a) Middle Finger Measurement: When the middle finger is flexed, the distance between the radial ends of the two interphalangeal creases of the patient's middle finger is considered one cun. (pronounced chun).

b) Thumb Measurement: The width of the interphalangeal joint of the patient's thumb is considered to be one cun.

c) Four-Finger Measurement: When the four fingers (index, middle, ring and little fingers) are kept close together, the width of them on the level of the proximal interphalangeal crease of the middle finger is taken as three cun. (See Figure 3-1.)

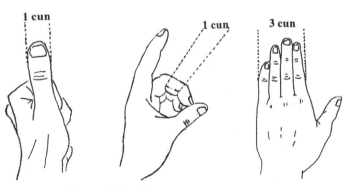

FIGURE 3-1 THE CUN AS A UNIT OF MEASUREMENT

When locating acupoints, this method should be used in combination with some simple moveable landmarks based on bone proportional measurement; this will help to increase your accuracy in locating acupoints.

Keep in mind that a practitioner's cun is not always equal to that of the patient's. So, before measuring and trying to calculate exactly where an acupoint is located, look at the difference in size between your finger and that of the patient. The cun must be that of the patient's in order to locate acupoints accurately. Moreover, because the exact acupoint is the center in which energy from that meridian has converged, accuracy in locating points is essential.

Bone Proportional Measurement

This method for locating acupoints uses joints as the main landmarks to measure the length and width of various portions of the human body. The proportional measurement of various portions of the human body is defined in the Miraculous Pivot (Ling Shu – an important reference guide for TCM practitioners) and is considered to be the basis for locating acupoints. This method is used in combination with the modified methods introduced by acupuncturists throughout the ages.

The length between two joints is divided into several equal portions. Each portion is measured as a cun (TCM measurement) and 10 portions as one chi (See Table 2-1). For an illustration showing the bone proportional measurements of the head and face, see Figure 3-2.

Major Surface Anatomical Landmarks on the Head and Face

This is a method that is used to determine the location of acupoints on the basis of anatomical landmarks on the body surface. These landmarks are divided into two classifications: Fixed Landmarks and Movable Landmarks.

The fixed landmarks include the prominences and depressions formed by joints and muscles. For instance, Zanzhu (UB 2) lies at the medial end of the eyebrow; Yintang (EX-HN 3) lies midway between the eyebrows. Several points are easily found because we have these landmarks to use as aids.

The movable landmarks refer to the clefts, depressions, wrinkles, or protuberances appearing on the joints, muscles, tendons, and skin during motion. For example, Tinggong (SI 19) lies between the tragus (gristle mound in front of ear hole), and the mandibular joint (jaw bone hinge), where a depression is formed when the mouth is slightly open. In order to find the movable landmarks, we must move a part of the body.

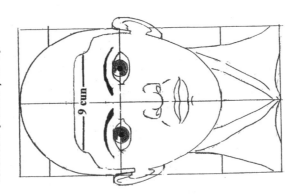

Between the corners of the forehead (Touwei, ST 8)

From Yintang (EX-HN3) to the midpoint of the anterior hairline

From the midpoint of the anterior hairline to the midpoint of the posterior hairline

From the point below the spinous process of the 7th cervical vertebra (Dazhui, DU14) to the midpoint of the posterior hairline

Between the bilateral mastoid processes

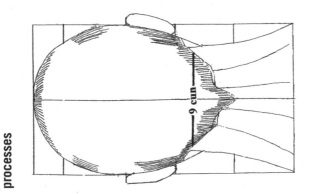

FIGURE 3-2 BONE PROPORTIONAL MEASUREMENTS

Origin and End Points	Portion (cun)	Directional	Remarks
From the midpoint of the anterior hairline to the midpoint of the posterior hairline	12	Longitudinal	Used for measuring the longitudinal distance of the points on the head
From Yintang (EX-HN 3) to the midpoint of the anterior hairline	3	Longitudinal	Used for measuring the longitudinal distance of points on the anterior and posterior hairline and head
From the point below the spinous process of the seventh cervical vertebra (Dazhui (GV (Du) 14) to the midpoint of the posterior hairline	3	Longitudinal	
From Yintang (EX-HN 3) to the midpoint of the anterior hairline, and then to the point below the spinous process of the seventh cervical vertebra (Dazhui (GV (Du) 14)	18	Longitudinal	
Between the corners of the forehead (Touwei, ST 8)	9	Transverse	Used for measuring the transverse distance of points on the anterior part of the head
Between the bilateral mastoid processes	9	Transverse	Used for measuring the transverse distance of the points on the posterior part of the head

TABLE 3-1 BONE PROPORTIONAL MEASUREMENT

CHAPTER 4

Terminology of Anatomical Directions

The descriptions of point locations use the following anatomical terminology in Figure 4-1 (following page).

Anatomical Directions

The following terminology is used to describe acupuncture point locations:

Anterior - At or nearer to the front

Posterior - At or nearer to the back

Superior - Towards the head or upper part

Inferior - Towards the lower part or away from the head

Medial - Nearer the midline

Lateral - Away from the midline

Proximal - Nearer to the attachment of an extremity to the body

Distal - Away from the attachment of an extremity to the body

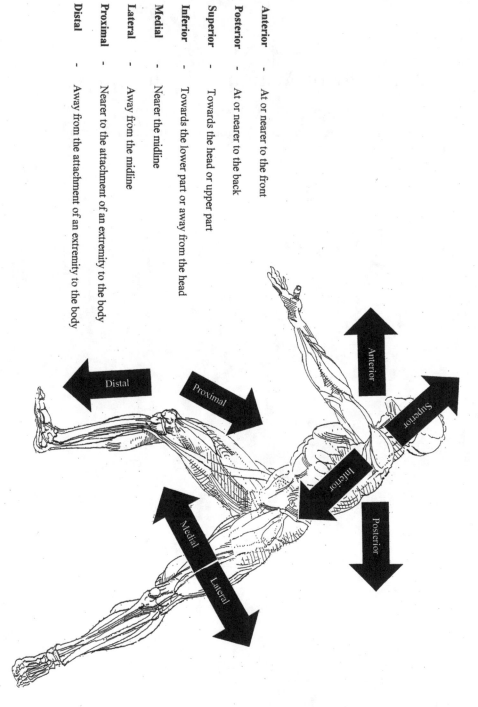

FIGURE 4-1 TERMINOLOGY OF ANATOMICAL DIRECTIONS

CHAPTER 5

Main Acupoints in Wu's Head Massage

The following 40 points are used in Wu's Head Massage. The order of the points approximates their use in the massage movements. Practice by locating these points on yourself. You will know by feel when they are found. They are sensitive, and often the fingertips feel a slight depression. Remember that points not on the midline are bilateral (found in pairs) so locate and practice accordingly.

Acupoint Name/Location	Massage Movements
1) Shenting (GV (Du) 24) Spirit Court (shen: spirit, ting: court, palace, hall—Face is the "court of spirit", the brain is the palace of spirit) Location: 0.5 cun directly above the midpoint of the anterior hairline	#1. Kneading and Pressing Zanzhu (UB 2) #36. Finger Combing and Wiping the Forehead
2) Zanzhu (UB 2) Bamboo Gathering (zan (pronounced caun): to gather, zhu: bamboo 6) 36)—A bundle of bamboo looks like eyebrow) Location: On the medial extremity of the eyebrow, at the supraorbital notch	#1. Kneading and Pressing Zanzhu (UB 2) #2. Wiping Forehead Meridians (Alternately) #6. Scraping the Eyebrows #36. Finger Combing and Wiping the Forehead
3) Yintang (EX-HN 3) Abundant Hall (yin: abundant, tang: meeting place, hall) Location: Midway between the medial end of the two eyebrows	#1. Kneading and Pressing Zanzhu (UB 2) #2. Wiping Forehead Meridians (Alternately) #3. Wiping the Forehead #36. Finger Combing and Wiping the Forehead
4) Yuyao (EX-HN 4) Fish Waist (yu: fish, yao: waist, kidneys) Location: At the midpoint of the eyebrow	#2. Wiping Forehead Meridians (Alternately) #4. Kneading and Pressing Yuyao (EX-HN 4) #36. Finger Combing and Wiping the Forehead
5) Sizhukong (SJ 23) Silk Bamboo Hole (si: silk, zhu: bamboo, kong: empty, hole) Location: In the depression at the lateral end of the eyebrow	#2. Wiping Forehead Meridians (Alternately) #5. Kneading and Pressing Sizhukong (SJ 23) #6. Scraping the Eyebrows #36. Finger Combing and Wiping the Forehead
6) Taiyang (EX-HN 5) Sun Location: In the depression about 1 cun posterior to the midpoint between the lateral end of the eyebrow and outer canthus	#3. Wiping the Forehead #28. Kneading the Temple—Taiyang (EX-HN 5)

Acupoint Name/Location	Massage Movements
7) Jingming (UB 1) Bright Eyes (jing: eye, pupil, ming: bright) Location: In the depression superior to the inner canthus—In the medial part of the eyelid crease	#7. Wiping the Eyeball #26. Stroking Jingming #27. Downward Squeezing of the Nose
8) Chengqi (ST 1) Tear Container (cheng: to contain, carry, gi: tears treats excessive eye watering due to wind) Location: With the eyes looking straight forward, the point is directly below the pupil, between the eyeball and the infraorbital ridge	#7. Wiping the Eyeball
9) Sibai (ST 2) Four Whites (si: four, bai: white, four whites of eye) Location: One cun below pupil, in the depression on infraorbital ridge—when looking straight ahead, one cun below pupil center	#7. Wiping the Eyeball
10) Tongziliao (GB 1) Pupil Bone Hole (tong: pupil, zi: noun/suffix, liao: bone hole) Location: 0.5 cun lateral to the outer canthus (where upper and lower lids meet) in the depression on the lateral side of the orbit	#7. Wiping the Eyeball
11) Yingxiang (LI 20) Welcome Fragrance (ying: to welcome, xiang: fragrance) Location: In the nasolabial groove, at the level of midpoint of the nostril flair	#8. Kneading and Pressing Yingxiang (LI 20) #26. Stroking Jingming #27. Downward Squeezing of the Nose
12) Dicang (ST 4) Earth Granary (di: earth, cang: granary, storehouse, like a granary because it receives food) Location: About 0.4 cun lateral to the corner of the mouth and vertically inferior to pupil when looking straight ahead	#9. Kneading and Pressing Dicang (ST 4) #26. Stroking Jingming
13) Daying (ST 5) Great Reception (da: great, large, ying: to welcome) Location: in the groove-like depression on the mandible ridge (jaw) appearing when the teeth are clenched. Anterior to the masseter attachment (jaw muscle) and level with mandible angle (jaw corner)	#10. Pressing Specific Acupressure Points
14) Jiache (ST 6) Jaw Bone (jia: jaw, che: vehicle, chariot Vehicle because it carries the teeth) Location: One finger-breadth anterior and superior to the mandible angle where major masseter attaches at the prominence of the muscle when the teeth are clenched	#10. Pressing Specific Acupressure Points
15) Xiaguan (ST 7) Below the Joint (xia: below, lower, guan: joint, hinge) Location: At the lower border of zygomatic arch, in the depression anterior to the condylar process of the mandible (jaw hinge). This point is located with the mouth closed	#10. Pressing Specific Acupressure Points

Acupoint Name/Location	Massage Movements
16) Tinghui (GB 2) Auditory Convergence (ting: to hear, hui: to converge) Location: Anterior to the intertragic notch, at the posterior border of the condylar process of the mandible. Just in front and below the tragus (gristly ridge in front of ear hole). The point is located with the mouth open	#10. Pressing Specific Acupressure Points
17) Tinggong (SI 19) Auditory Palace (ting: to hear, gong: palace) Location: Level to the center of the ear tragus, between the tragus and the condylar process (jaw hinge) in the depression formed when the mouth is open. Approximately 0.5 cun directly above Tinghui	#10. Pressing Specific Acupressure Points
18) Ermen (SJ 21) Ear Gate (er: ear, men: gate, door) Location: With mouth open, between ear cartilage and condylar process Level with top edge of the tragus. Approximately 0.5 cun directly above Tinggong (SI 19)	#10. Pressing Specific Acupressure Points
19) Lianquan (CV (Ren) 23) Ridge Spring (lian: ridge, corner, quan: spring) Location: Above the Adam's Apple, in the depression of the upper border of the hyoid bone. On the center line where under the chin meets the neck	#11. Kneading and Pressing Chengjiang (CV (Ren) 24)
20) Chengjiang (CV (Ren) 24) Sauce Receptacle (cheng: to receive, jiang: sauce) Location: In the depression in the center of the mentolabial groove; the crease in the middle of the chin	#11. Kneading and Pressing Chengjiang (CV (Ren) 24)
21) Baihui (GV (Du) 20) Hundred Convergences (bai: hundred, hui: meeting—six Yang meridians converge here) Location: On the midline of the head, approximately on the midpoint of the line connecting the apex of the two ears. Seven cun superior to the midpoint of the anterior hairline	#10. Pressing Specific Acupressure Points #13. Scalp Sweeping Method (Right Side of Head) #32. Digital Pressing Baihui (GV (Du) 20)
22) Shuaigu (GB 8) Valley Lead (shuai: to lead, gu: valley) Location: Superior to the apex of the ear, 1.5 cun within the hairline. In the depression of the temple aspect	#13. Scalp Sweeping Method (Right Side of Head) #14. Scalp Finger-Combing Method (Right Side)
23) Renying (ST 9) Man's Prognosis (ren: person, ying: to expect) Location: Level with the tip of the Adam's apple, just on course of the common carotid artery, on the anterior border of sternocleidomastoid (front to side neck muscle)	#12. Stroking the Right Side of the Neck #18 Stroking the Left Side of the Neck

Acupoint Name/Location	Massage Movements
24) Futu (LI 18) Protuberance Assistant (fu: to aid, tu: protuberance) Location: On the lateral side of the neck, 3 cun outside on the level with tip of the Adam's Apple, in the center of sternocleidomastoid	#12. Stroking the Right Side of the Neck #18 Stroking the Left Side of the Neck
25) Quepen (ST 12) Empty Basin (que: empty, vacant, pen: basin) Location: In the midpoint of the supraclavicular fossa (collar bone) 4 cun lateral to Ren Meridian	#12. Stroking the Right Side of the Neck #18 Stroking the Left Side of the Neck
26) Shuigou (GV (Du) 26) Water Trough (shui: water, gou: trough, ditch) Location: A little way above the midpoint of the philtrum (vertical groove above upper lip) near nostrils	#25. Stroking Shuigou (GV (Du) 26) (Both Sides of the Philtrum) #18 Stroking the Left Side of the Neck
27) Fengchi (GB 20) Wind Pool (feng: wind, chi: pool, pond—wind pathogens collect in this spot) Location: In the depression between the upper portion of sternocleidomastoideus and musculus trapezius, on the same level with Fengfu (GV (Du) 16) Where the side neck muscle meets the back neck muscle near the base of skull	#30. Digital Pressing Fengchi (GB 20)
28) Suliao (GV (Du) 25) White Bone Hole (su: pure, white (lung), liao: bone hole) Location: On the tip of the nose	#27. Downward Squeezing of the Nose
29) Yifeng (SJ 17) Wind Screen (yi: screen, feng: wind—dispels wind) Location: Behind the earlobe, in the depression between the mandible and the mastoid process	#31. Digital Pressing Yifeng (SJ 17)
30) Sishencong (EX-HN 1) Four Spirits (si: four, shen: spirit, cong: smart) Location: A group of 4 points at the head vertex, 1 cun posterior, anterior and lateral to Baihui (GV (Du) 20)	#33. Digital Pressing Sishencong (EX-HN 1)
31) Shangxing (GV (Du) 23) Upper Star (shang: upper, xing: star) Location: 1 cun directly above the midpoint of the anterior hairline	#36. Finger Combing and Wiping the Forehead
32) Quchai (UB 4) Deviating Turn (qui: crooked, cha: difference—where the Urinary Bladder meridian deviates laterally) Location: 1.5 cun lateral to the head midline and 0.5 cun superior to anterior hairline	#36. Finger Combing and Wiping the Forehead
3) Toulinqi (GB 15) Head Overlooking Tears (tou: head, lin: to overlook, qi: tear) Location: Directly above GB14, 0.5 cun superior to front hairline, 2.25 cun lateral to head midline	#36. Finger Combing and Wiping the Forehead

Acupoint Name/Location	Massage Movements
34) Touwei (ST 8) Head Corner (tou: head, wei: corner) Location: 0.5 cun superior to front hairline, 4.5 cun lateral to midline, level with GV 24	#36. Finger Combing and Wiping the Forehead
35) Fengfu (GV (Du) 16) Wind Mansion (feng: wind, fu: mansion) Location: 1 cun directly above the midpoint of the posterior hairline, directly below the external occipital protuberance, in depression between trapezius (back neck muscle) of both sides	#45. Kneading and Grasping the Neck Tendons
36) Tianding (LI 17) Celestial Tripod (tian: heaven, celestial ding: ancient Chinese cooking vessel. Neck holding the head is like a tripod) Location: On the lateral side of the neck, on the posterior border of sternocleidomastoid, one cun below Neck-Futu	#12. Stroking the Right Side of the Neck #18 Stroking the Left Side of the Neck #47. Pushing and Pressing the Sternocleidomastoid Muscle
37) Dazhui (GV (Du) 14) Great Hammer (da: big, zhui: hammer Chinese call vertebrae "spine hammer") Location: Below the spinous process of the seventh cervical vertebra, approximately at the level of the shoulders	#49. Kneading and Pressing Dazhui (GV (Du) 14)
38) Jianjing (GB 21) Shoulder Well (jian: shoulder, jing: well) Location: Midway between Dazhui and the acromion, at the highest point of the shoulder	#50. Rolling and Pressing the Neck
39) Quanliao (SI 18) Cheek Bone Hole (quan: cheekbone liao: bone hole) Location: Directly below the outer canthus, in the depression on the lower border of zygoma (cheek bone arch)	#25. Stroking Shuigou (GV (Du) 26) (Both Sides of the Philtrum)
40) Tiantu (CV (Ren) 22) Celestial Chimney (tian: heavens, tu:chimney—windpipe is like a chimney) Location: In the center of the suprasternal fossa. The midline depression where the two collarbones almost meet	#12. Stroking the Right Side of the Neck #18 Stroking the Left Side of the Neck

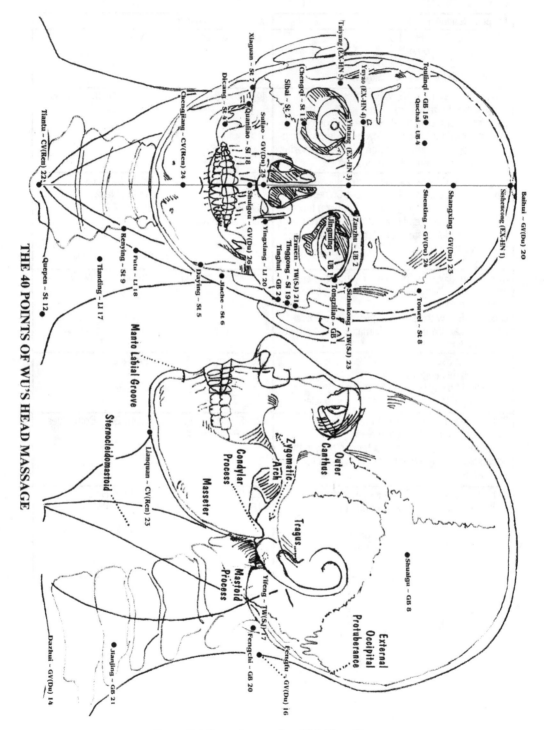

THE 40 POINTS OF WU'S HEAD MASSAGE

FIGURE 5-1 FORTY ACUPOINTS IN WU'S HEAD MASSAGE

PART III
Stimulation Areas on Face and Head

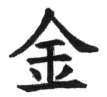

CHAPTER 6

The Face's Stimulation Areas

As mentioned earlier in this book, more than 2,000 years ago, the earliest recorded medical text collection in China was *The Yellow Emperor's Canon of Internal Medicine* (Wu Se Pian, one of the treatises of Lin Shu Jing). This text systematically expounded that various areas on the face (referred to as stimulation areas) governed different organs and parts of the body. From the color changes in these stimulation areas combined with the type of pulse found during diagnosis, one could infer the occurrence, development, change, and anticipation of diseases. In this chapter these stimulation areas are organized as Face, Head, and Ear

The face's stimulation areas, according to Wu Se Pian and through intensive and vast clinical experience were recorded, and then divided into Six Major Stimulation Areas. To fully understand the stimulation areas and their locations, it is beneficial to have some background in basic anatomy.

Stimulation Area 1. This area is the Upper-Jiao, from the horizontal line of the eye-orbital to the anterior hairline (the frontal and ocular zone).

Stimulation Area 2. The next are is part of the Middle-Jiao, from the horizontal line of the nostril wing of the nose to the horizontal line of the eye-orbital (the nasal zone and the zone of zygoma (cheekbones).

Stimulation Area 3. The next area is the Lower-Jiao, located below the horizontal line of the wing of the nose (the oral zone and the zone of medial border of the cheek).

Stimulation Area 4. This area is the spine and the back, located in the auditory zone.

Stimulation Area 5. This area is allocated to the upper limbs, the zone of zygoma.

Stimulation Area 6. This area is designated to the lower limbs and is located in the zone of the cheek and the oral zone and mandible.

Exact Locations and Indications of Stimulation Areas

1. Upper-Jiao (also referred to as the Upper Burner)

Begins at the horizontal line of the eye orbital to the anterior hairline, and includes the following:

a. Face and Head Area
Location: on the forehead.
Indication: diseases of the head or face.

b. Throat Area
Location: between the face-head area and the lung area, above the area between the eyebrows (called "Que Shang").
Indication: diseases of the throat.

c. Lung Area
Location: at the middle of the line connecting the medial ends of the two eyebrows.
Indication: diseases of the lungs.

d. Heart Area
Location: at the middle of the line connecting the two inner canthuses at the lowest place at the bridge of the nose.
Indication: diseases of the heart.

e. Breast and Nipple Area
Location: slightly above the inner canthus, between the heart area and inner canthus, in the depression of the exterior border of the bridge of the nose.
Indication: abnormal lactation, and eye diseases.

2. Middle-Jiao (also referred to as the Middle Burner)

From the horizontal line of the wing (nostril) of the nose to the horizontal line of the eye-orbital (The nasal zone and the zone of medial border of the zygomatic bone)

a. Liver Area
Location: the crossing point between the nasal medial lines connecting the two regions of zygoma.
Indication: diseases of the liver.

b. Spleen Area
Location: slightly above the center of the upper border of the apex of the nose, (called "Mian Wang").
Indication: diseases of the spleen.

c. Biliary Area
Location: at both sides of the liver area, directly below the inner canthus.
Indication: diseases of the gallbladder.

d. Stomach Area
Location: at both sides of the spleen area, slightly above the center of the wing

(nostril) of the nose, directly below the biliary area.
Indication: diseases of the stomach.

  e. Small Intestine Area
Location: at the medial border of the zygomatic bone and the outside of the midpoint connecting the stomach area and the biliary area.
Indication: diseases of the small intestine.

  f. Large Intestine Area
Location: the center of the face, directly below the small intestine area, at the crossing point between the line of the small intestine area and the stomach area.
Indication: diseases of the large intestine.

3. Lower-Jiao (also referred to as the Lower Burner)

Below the horizontal line of the wing of the nose (The oral zone and the zone of the medial border of the cheek)

  a. Urinary Bladder, Uterus and Genital Area.
Location: at the nasolabial sulcus (philtrum).
Indication: diseases of urinary bladder, uterus and genitals.

  b. Kidney Area
Location: at both sides of the large intestine area, in the horizontal line of the wing (nostril) of the nose.
Indication: diseases of the kidney.

  c. Umbilical Area
Location: at the cheek region, below the kidney area.
Indication: umbilical diseases.

4. Spine and Back (includes the Auditory Zone)

  a. The Spine and Back Area
Location: anterior to the tragus, at the middle between the medial aspect of the tragus and the mandible joint.
Indication: pain in the spine and back.

5. Upper Limbs (includes the Zone of Zygoma)

  a. Shoulder Area
Location: at the cheekbone and below the outer canthus.
Indication: bursitis, arthritis, injury.

  b. Arm Area
Location: runs downward along the zygomatic bone, posterior to the shoulder area, and below the border of the zygomatic bone.
Indication: arthritis, injury.

  c. Hand Area
Location: below the arm area.
Indication: arthritis, injury.

6. Lower Limbs (Zone of the Cheek, Oral Zone, and Mandible)

a. Groin Area
Location: 0.5 can lateral to the angle of the mouth, where the lips meet.
Indication: diseases of the mouth and lips, and pain in the groin area.

b. Thigh Area
Location: at the boundary between the upper and middle 1/3 of the line connecting the auricular lobe and the angle of the mandible.
Indication: diseases of the thigh.

c. Knee Area
Location: at the boundary between the lower and middle 1/3 of the line connecting the auricular lobe and the angle of the mandible.
Indication: diseases of the knee.

d. Knee and Patella Area
Location: at the muscular protuberance when the teeth are clenched, anterior and superior to the angle of the mandible.
Indication: diseases of the knee or patella.

e. Tibia Area
Location: anterior to the angle of the mandible, it is at the anterior and lower area of the knee.
Indication: diseases of the tibia region.

f. Foot Area
Location: at the anterior and lower areas of the tibia.
Indication: diseases of the foot.

The Distribution Stimulation Areas were first introduced thousands of years ago, but it is only now, that a visual depiction of these areas has been created. Dr. Wu's intention has been to make this theory and massage therapy accessible to everyone.

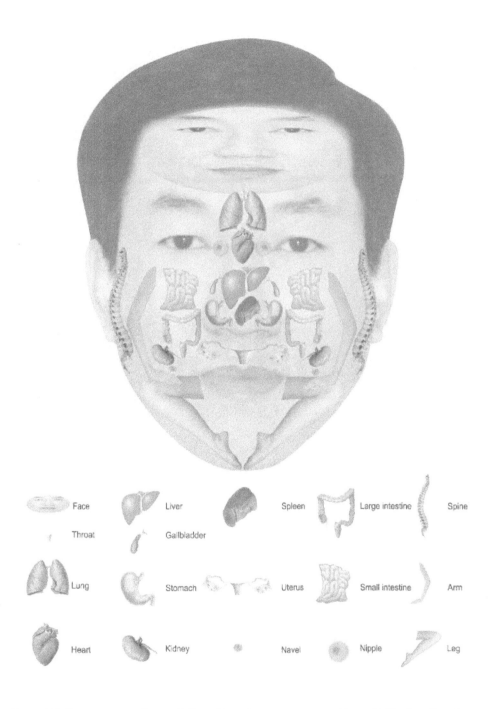

FIGURE 6-1 DISTRIBUTION OF ORGANS & BODY PARTS AS DISCUSSED IN THE *HUANG DI NEI JING* (*THE YELLOW EMPEROR'S CANON OF INTERNAL MEDICINE*)

CHAPTER 7

The Head's Stimulation Areas

The Head Stimulation Areas have been divided into 3 parts:
- Lateral Side of the Head (side).
- Anterior Side of the Head (front).
- Posterior Side of the Head (back).

Each area is responsible for different parts of the brain, body parts and functions.

There are two standard lines that are used to divide the stimulation areas of the head. One is called the Antero-Posterior Midline, the other is the Eyebrow-Occiput Line.

Stimulation Areas of the Lateral Side of the Head

1) Motor Area

Location: The point 0.5 cm posterior to the midpoint of the Antero-Posterior Midline is the upper point, and the intersection of the Eyebrow-Occiput Line, the anterior border of the natural line of the hair at the temple, is the lower point. The connecting line between these two points is the Motor Area. The area is subdivided into five equal parts.

a) the upper 1/5 is the Lower Limb and Trunk Motor Area

b) the middle 2/5 is the Upper Limb Motor Area

c) the lower 2/5 is the Facial Motor Area.

Indications: the upper 1/5 of the Motor Area is responsible for contra-lateral paralysis of the lower limbs; the middle 2/5 for contra-lateral paralysis of the upper limbs; and the lower 2/5 for contra-lateral central facial paralysis, motor aphasis, salivation, and dysphonia.

2) Sensory Area

Location: The parallel line, 1.5 can behind the Motor Area, is where the Sensory Area is located. The upper 1/5 of this area houses the Lower Limbs, Head and Trunk Sensory Area; the middle 2/5 is the Upper Limb Sensory Area; and the lower 2/5 is the Facial Sensory Area.

Indication: the upper 1/5 of the Sensory Area is responsible for contra-lateral pain, pain of the leg, numbness, paresthesia, occipital headache, pain in the nape region and tinnitus; the middle 2/5 for contra-lateral upper limb pain, numbness and paresthesia; and the lower 1/5 for contra-lateral facial numbness, migraines, trigeminal neuralgia, toothache, and temporomandibular arthritis.

3) Chorea Trembling Controlled Area

Location: the parallel line, 1.5 cm in front of the Motor Area

Indications: chorea, Parkinson's Disease, (If the symptom is unilateral, massage the Contrary Stimulation Area. If bilateral, massage bilaterally.)

4) Vertigo-Auditory Area

Location: a 4-cm horizontal, straight line located on the site, 1.5 cm directly above the Auricular Apex.

Indication: Tinnitus, hypoacusis, vertigo, auditory vertigo.

5) Second Speech Area

Location: a 3-cm straight line, starting from the point 2 cm posterior and inferior to the parietal tubercle, parallel to the anteroom posterior midline.

Indication: nominal aphasia.

6) Third Speech Area

Location: 4 cm horizontal line running backwards from the midpoint of the Vertigo-Auditory Area.

Indication: sensory aphasia.

7) Usage Area

Location: Take the parietal tubercle as a starting point; draw a vertical line from that point. At the same time, draw two other lines from the point, one running forward and the other running backwards, at 40-degree angles with the vertical line, each of the three lines being 3 cm long.

Indication: apraxia.

See massage movements 13, 14, 15, 16, 19, 20, 21, 22, 41, 44 of Wu's Head Massage Sequence (described in Chapter 9) (See Figures 7-1 and 7-2).

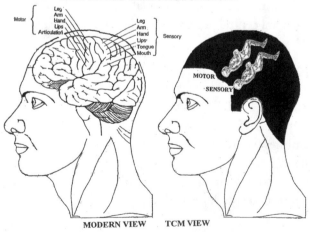

MOTOR AND SENSORY FUNCTION

FIGURE 7-1 MOTOR AND SENSORY FUNCTIONS

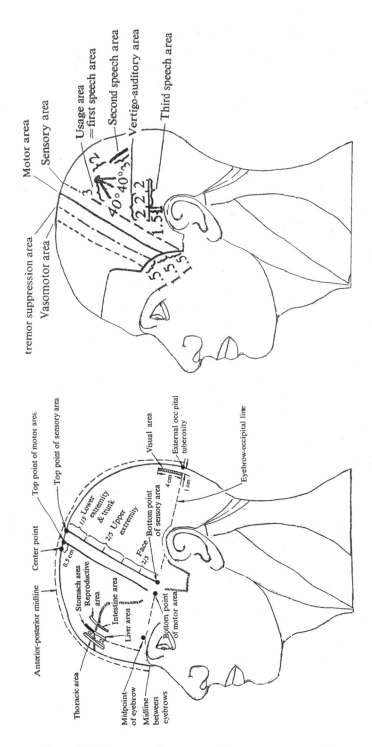

FIGURE 7-2 STIMULATION AREAS ON THE FRONT AND SIDE OF THE HEAD

Stimulation Areas of the Anterior Side of the Head

8) Gastric Area

Location: Take the hair margin directly above the pupil as a starting point; draw a 2-cm straight line upwards, parallel to the Antero-Posterior Midline.

Indication: gastric pain, epigastric discomfort.

9) Thoracic Area

Location: Midway between the Gastric Area and the Antero-Posterior Midline. Taking the hair margin as the midpoint, draw a 4-cm straight line, parallel to the Antero-Posterior Midline.

Indication: chest pain, chest stuffiness, palpitations, coronary and artery insufficiency, asthma, and hiccups.

10) Reproduction Area

Location: Draw a 2-cm straight line from the frontal angle upward, parallel to the Antero- Posterior Midline.

Indication: functional uterine bleeding, pelvic inflammation, leukorrhagia. prolapse of the uterus and other areas prone to prolapse, may be treated in association with the Foot Motor Sensory Area.

See massage movements 2, 3, 29, 34, 35, 36, 37, 38, 39, 40 of Wu's Head Massage Sequence (described in Chapter 9) (See Figure 7-3).

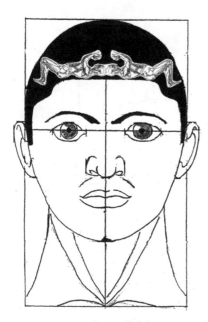 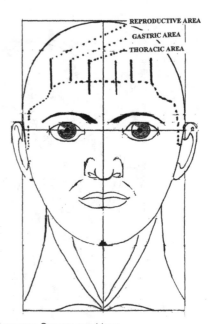

FIGURE 7-3 STIMULATION AREAS OF ANTERIOR SIDE OF THE HEAD

Stimulation Areas of the Posterior Side of the Head

11) Foot Motor Sensory Area

Location: Draw two 3-cm straight lines backwards and parallel to the Antero-Posterior Midline. Their starting points are 1 cm bilateral to the midpoint of the midline.

Indication: contra-lateral lower limb pain, numbness, paralysis, acute lumbar sprain, cerebro-cortical polyuria, nocturia, prolapse of the uterus.

12) Optic Area

Location: Draw a 4-cm straight line upwards, and parallel to the Antero-Posterior Midline, 1 cm evenly beside the external occipital protuberance.

Indication: cerebro-cortical visual disturbance.

13) Balance Area

Location: Draw a 4-cm straight line downwards, and parallel to the Antero-Posterior Midline, 3.5 cm evenly beside the external occipital protuberance.

Indication: equilibrium disturbance caused by cerebellum disease.

See massage movements 30, 32, 33, 42, 45 of Wu's Head Massage Sequence (described in Chapter 9) (See Figure 7-4).

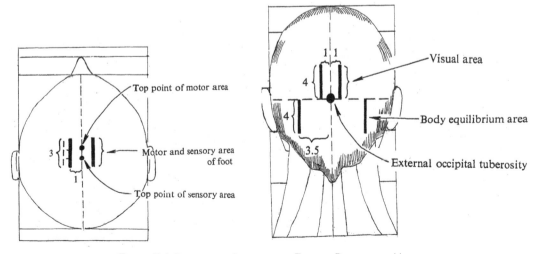

FIGURE 7-4 STIMULATION AREAS ON THE TOP AND BACK OF THE HEAD

Stimulation Areas of the Ear

In TCM, the ear is also considered to be a blueprint of the body. Many practitioners of TCM use auricular acupuncture to treat many illnesses and diseases. In a WHM treatment, we do a light massage on the auricular region.

Distribution and Indications of Auricular Points

An easy way to remember how the various body parts are distributed on the ear, is to imagine a fetus curled up on the surface of the ear. The placement of the body areas on the auricle is just like a fetus with the head downward and the buttocks upward.

Distribution of Auricular Points

Points on the lobule: related to the head and facial regions

Points on the scapha: related to the upper limbs

Points on the antihelixes and its two crura: related to the trunk and lower limbs

Points on the cavum and cymba conchae: related to the internal organs

Points arranged as a ring around the helix crus: related to the digestive tract

Indication: Stimulate the auricular points related to the parts of the body that need treatment, or are diseased or ill.

See massage movements 17 and 23 of Wu's Head Massage Sequence (described in Chapter 9) (See Figure 7-5).

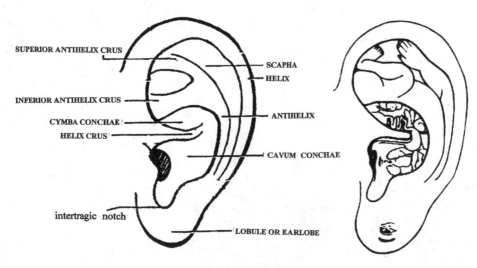

FIGURE 7-5 THE EAR

PART IV
Wu's Head Massage

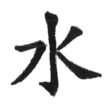

CHAPTER 8

Manipulations

Wu's Head Massage requires accurate point location and correct massage technique. The following manipulations are the 'tools' of the practitioner. Doing these manipulations correctly and often is the key to success. Practicing on your thigh while sitting, for example, lets you assess the effects of your touch. Over time and with effort, these manipulations become smooth and natural. The effects of these manipulations are given in Traditional Chinese Medical terms. Do not be alarmed. This is a journey, and as with any journey, knowledge and insight will deepen over time.

Kneading Manipulation

This manipulation is performed by slowly and softly kneading the therapeutic region to and fro with the fingers, the bottom of the palm, the ball of the thumb (major thenar eminence), or the tip of the elbow. The kneading manipulation can be divided into middle-finger kneading manipulation, thumb-kneading manipulation, palm-root kneading manipulation, major-thenar kneading manipulation, and elbow-kneading manipulation depending on what is used and according to what is treated. In this manipulation, the operator is in a sitting position. He presses the treatment region with his middle finger, thumb tip, palm root, and with the coordination of his shoulder, elbow, forearm and wrist joint, does annular rotation within a narrow range. This causes the skin of the treated region to rotate slowly and softly so that a soft, light, and

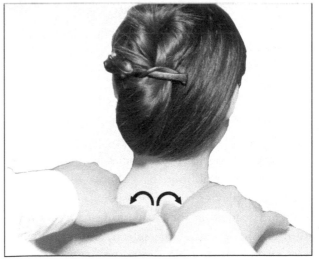

FIGURE 8-1 KNEADING MANIPULATION

slow internal rubbing is produced between the skin and the internal soft tissue. The whole manipulation emphasizes softness and the range of kneading, and rotating should be gradually extended, and the force gradually increased. The operating hand should be fixed on the treated region without any rubbing or slipping on the skin surface. The frequency is about 100-160 times per minute. The impact of kneading is light, soft and slow, but deep and thorough. Warmth can be created in the deep layer of the tissue by the internal rubbing caused by kneading. Kneading manipulation has the following effects: soothing chest oppression and regulating the flow of Qi, strengthening the spleen and regulating the stomach, promoting blood circulation to remove blood stasis, reducing swelling and alleviating pain, expelling pathogenic wind and cold, promoting the flow of Qi by warming the channel, tranquilizing the mind, and relieving spasms, etc.

Rubbing Manipulation

The technique performed by rhythmically rubbing the working surface in a circular motion with the palm or the pads of the practitioner's fingers is called rubbing. Palm-rubbing or finger rubbing is usually done by the practitioner in a sitting position. He lowers his shoulder and drops his elbow with his forearm in a prone position and his palm facing downwards. In palm-rubbing manipulation, the practitioner slightly flexes his wrist with the whole palm pressing on the therapeutic part. In finger-rubbing manipulation, he flexes his wrist about 160 degrees and lifts up his palm transferring power to the finger surface. With the cooperative motion of his shoulder, elbow, and the palmar surface as the power center, the practitioner begins a circular rotation in either a clockwise or a counterclockwise direction. Its frequency should be moderate, even, and steady, about 100-120 cycles per minute. Rubbing has the effects of relieving the depressed

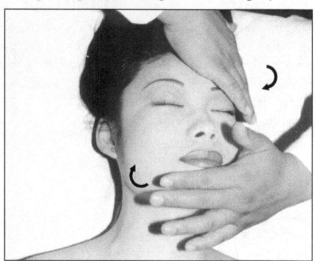

FIGURE 8-2 RUBBING MANIPULATION

liver and regulating the circulation of Qi, warming the middle jiao and regulating the stomach, invigorating the spleen, promoting digestion, removing stagnant food and encouraging the intestines to move.

Grasping Manipulation

Grasping manipulation is performed by symmetrically and slowly lifting and squeezing the therapeutic region and meanwhile holding and twisting, kneading and pinching it with the operator's thumb and index finger and middle finger or with five fingers.

Using the thumb index and middle finger is called three-fingers grasping, using all five, five-fingers grasping. In a sitting or standing position, the practitioner lowers his shoulder flexes his elbow about 90 degrees to 110 degrees with his thumb and fingers he holds the tendon or muscle bundle of the therapeutic part, lifts it up and meanwhile twirls and kneads it, and releases it after stimulating it several times. This is done repeatedly. During the operation, every movement should be coordinated rhythmical. The part being lifted and grasped is chiefly the cord tissue such as tendon, ligament, and muscle bundle of layers of the body. Holding the skin or digging and nipping the treated region with finger nails should be avoided in case it causes discomfort or pain. This stimulation is deep and heavy but the manipulation is soft. It has the following effects: restoring consciousness, relieving wind and cold, relaxing muscles and tendons to promote blood circulation, and relieving spasm and pain.

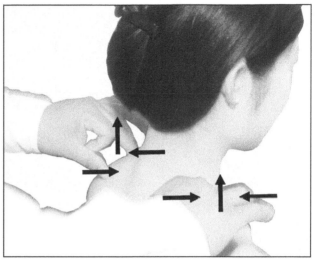

FIGURE 8-3 GRASPING MANIPULATION

This manipulation has the effects of relaxing muscles and tendons and activating the flow of Qi and blood in the channels and collaterals, promoting blood circulation to remove blood stasis, and regulating Qi and blood.

Patting Manipulation

Striking with the empty palm on the body surface is called patting or pat-hitting manipulation. The practitioner can be either in sitting or in standing position. The fingers are closed, joints are slightly flexed as to form an empty palm. The practitioner lifts up the hand, and pats down on the treated region with elastic and skillful strength. The hand bounces up right away to its initial position so as to perform the next patting. The stimulus of this therapy can be divided into light, intermediate and heavy types. The structure of this operation is similar to that of digital striking manipulation. This manipulation is mainly used on the shoulder and back, lower back, and the thigh. Light patting can also be used on thoracic-abdominal region and the head. Lasting and strong patting has the effect of sedation,

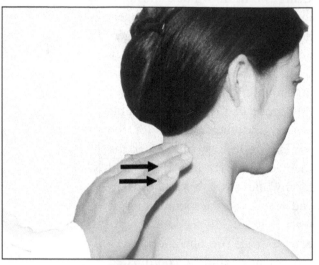

FIGURE 8-4 PATTING MANIPULATION

pain reduction, promoting blood circulation and removing blood stasis, strengthening the body, etc. Short and light patting has a mind and spirit calming effect and the effect of invigorating the nervous system, regulating the function of the stomach and intestines, soothing the chest oppression, and regulating the flow of Qi.

Tapping Manipulation

Using the back of fist, palm root, palm center, or the minor thenar eminence (palm muscles at the little finger side) to pound and hit the body surface is called tapping or striking manipulation.

Palm-tapping manipulation includes palm-center-striking and palm-root-tapping, the practitioner keeps the fingers combined, with the thumb in a natural flexed position, the wrist joint stretched backwards 45 degrees, and the protruding palm root directed at the treated region. In palm-center-striking, the doctor keeps the fingers combined with the thumb out of the way and the wrist and hand joints slightly flexed. This manipulation is similar to patting manipulation.

Minor thenar-hitting is also called "side-hitting" or "cut-beating." In this manipulation the

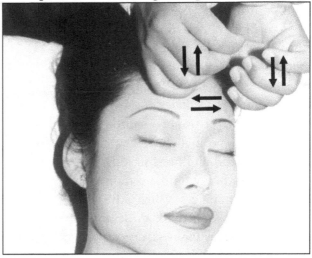

FIGURE 8-5 TAPPING MANIPULATION

practitioner opens the hands keeping the fingers combined and the forearm and the palm in a neutral position then beats the treated area rhythmically either with one or two hands, using the outside of the minor eminence to apply force. When tapping manipulation is employed, the force used should be decisive and swift. The tapping should be very short. In tapping the wrist should be relaxed, and blows are executed with a controlled elastic force so that the patient can feel relaxed and comfortable.

Pressing Manipulation

Pressing is done on the therapeutic region continuously with the practitioner's fingertip, palm, palm-root or the tip of his elbow, from lightly to heavily, shallowly to deeply. According to the different parts used, it can be divided into thumb-pressing manipulation or middle finger pressing manipulation.

The practitioner can adopt a sitting posture in light pressure manipulation, and standing posture in heavy pressure manipulation in order to generate force easily. The practitioner should breathe in a normal way (never hold the breath) and press steadily from light to heavy until a certain depth is attained. When the patient has experienced evident sensations such as soreness, distention, numbness and radiation, the practitioner keeps his hand on the area for about 5-10 minutes, then slowly lifts his hand up.

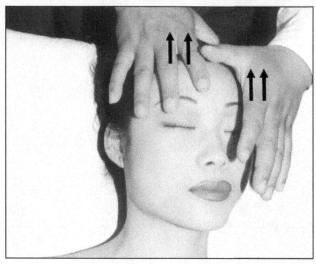

FIGURE 8-6 PRESSING MANIPULATION

This manipulation has the following effects: tranquilizing the mind and calming, relieving spasm and pain, reviving, relieving joint pain, removing obstruction in the channel, strengthening the tendon and muscles, etc.

Digital Pressing Manipulation

Digital pressing is the manipulation performed by heavily pressing the deep tissue layer with the operator's thumb or his middle finger tip, the index finger, or the joint of his flexed middle finger. It can be divided into thumb pressing, middle-finger-pressing, and finger joint pressing manipulations. This manipulation evolved from pressing manipulation, so there are similarities. The difference is that digital pressing has strong stimulation, so special attention should be paid to protecting the fingers. For example, in finger-pressing, the finger or thumb is reinforced at the joint by other fingers to avoid the sprain caused by sudden tiredness and softness of the joint, thus making the manipulation stable, solid and effective. This manipulation has a small and concentrated acting area, and the targeted layer is deep. It is applied to the indurate tissue of muscles or between bones or tenderness points and it has a positive effect of "treating pain with pain."

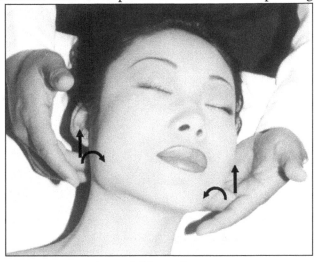

FIGURE 8-7 DIGITAL PRESSING

Holding-Twisting Manipulation

Grasping parts such as fingers and toes with the thumb and the forefinger and rolling- kneading to and fro with relative force is called holding-twisting manipulation. There are three ways of pinching the fingers and toes of the patient: with palmer side of the thumb, index or middle fingers: with palmer side of the thumb and the middle joint of the first index finger which is flexed into the shape of a bow. The holding-twisting should be dexterous and quick. A tacit agreement is needed between the acts of holding the thumb and fingers. In addition, the force used should be significant but even and moderate.

This manipulation is applied primarily to small joints of the fingers, toes, and fingertips. It has the function of lubricating joints, reducing swelling, alleviating pain,

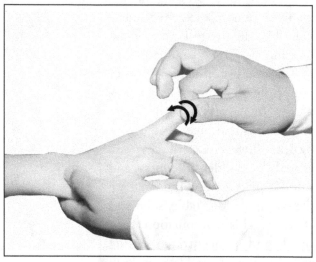

FIGURE 8-8 HOLDING-TWISTING MANIPULATION

and relaxing muscles and tendons to promote blood circulation, and is used mainly to treat symptoms of aching pain, swelling, uncontrolled flexing and stretching, and sprain of finger and toe joints. It may also be used as a supplementary manipulation to treat cervical joint problems, paralysis, and numbness of extremities. It can be done by operating repeatedly around the joints or moving slowly from the finger roots to tip while holding-twisting.

Wiping Manipulation

Wiping manipulation is performed by softly rubbing the skin of the affected part with the surface of one or two thumbs, up and down, or right and left, in a straight path. In two-hand wiping, if in one direction, the two hands should move along a straight line, and up and down alternatively; if in two directions, the two hands operate simultaneously. Frequency should be even, about 100-120 times per minute. The force used should be moderate, not too great to eliminate surface effect. To avoid skin scratches, a medium such as talc powder can be used. Wiping is a manipulation of lighter stimulus, mainly applied to head, face, five sense organs, and cervical part, which has the function of inducing resuscitation, tranquilizing the mind, restoring consciousness, improving vision,

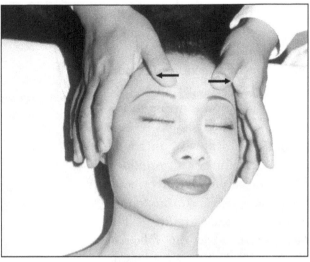

FIGURE 8-9 WIPING MANIPULATION

alleviating pain, and relaxing muscles and tendons to promote blood circulation. It is also used for symptoms of headache dizziness, facial paralysis, eye pressure, and neck pain and stiffness.

Traction and Counter-Traction Manipulation

The practitioner uses pulling-extending with much force in opposite directions on the upper and lower ends of joints longitudinally. This is called traction and counter-traction, or pulling or leading. The method is as follows; with one hand holding the proximal end of the operated joint and the other hand holding its distal end, the practitioner applies force simultaneously with both hands and uses traction and counter-traction to enlarge joint space. In the course of this manipulation, the force applied should be even lasting and slowly increased. Violent pulling is forbidden. Direction of pulling force should be applied with great care to joint deformity and rigidity. This manipulation has the following effects: with the function of restoring and treating injured soft tissues, reducing dislocated joints, enlarging joint spaces, relieving nerve compression, and treating adhesion.

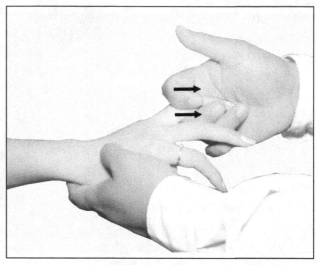

FIGURE 8-10 TRACTION AND COUNTER-TRACTION

CHAPTER 9

The Complete Wu's Head Massage Sequence

Preliminary Preparation

Immediately prior to beginning a Wu's Head Massage treatment, the practitioner should focus on three areas: the environment, themselves, and the patient. The therapist should also be aware of the contraindications for a WHM treatment.

The environment should be softly lit, free of harsh bright lights or direct sunlight. Soothing music or traditional Chinese music can greatly enhance the atmosphere.

The practitioner should remove rings or jewelry and sanitize their well-manicured hands. They should meditate briefly to reach a peaceful state, and adjust and regulate their breathing.

The patient should also remove any jewelry: necklaces, ear or nose rings, etc. Loose comfortable clothing is recommended with an open collar to allow access to the neck.

Contraindications for Giving a WHM Treatment

Do not do WHM under the following conditions:
- Head or facial dermal skin infections are present.
- Tumors of lesions are present.
- There is mental disturbance or agitation, preventing relaxation.
- Pregnancy with a history of miscarriage.

Wu's Head Massage can be done on women experiencing a health pregnancy, provided that only light pressure and stimulation are used.

Step-by-Step Instructions on Each Massage Movement

Now that you have an understanding of the basic principles and theories of Traditional Chinese Medicine (TCM), and Wu's Head Massage (WHM), you are ready to learn how to give a complete WHM treatment. Treatments last about 45 minutes in duration, depending on the needs and time constraints of the patient. What follows is a step-by-step guide to performing a full head massage treatment. Each massage movement is usually repeated 4-6 times. When a massage movement is done 4 times, the pressure on the first is light, the second heavier, the third heavier still, and the forth again light. The more practical experience the practitioner has, the more easily he or she can detect disharmony, blockage, and imbalances in the patient. Although a therapeutic massage, WHM also relieves stress and encourages relaxation. For most of the treatment, the patient is lying in a supine position, while the practitioner sits facing the crown of the head.

The 60 Movements of the Wu's Head Massage Sequence

Movement 1. Kneading and Pressing Zanzhu (UB 2)

Rest the tip of the thumb of one hand on Shenting (GV (Du) 24), while placing the pads of the index and middle fingers on Zanzhu (UB 2), kneading in a circular motion and pressing 4 to 6 times. You can also perform this same manipulation on Yintang (EX-HN 3), which is the midpoint between the eyebrows.

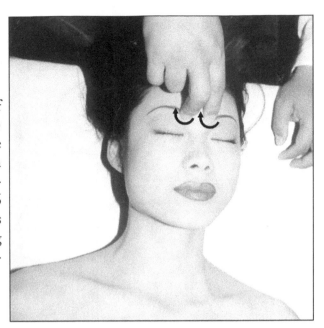

Movement 2. Wiping Forehead Meridians (Alternately)

With flattened thumbs, wipe the head in a straight line, alternating between the right and left thumb, all the way from Yintang (EX-HN 3) to the apex of the head. Then return to Zanzhu (UB 2) and wipe backwards/downwards again to the apex of the head. Repeat this same manipulation with Yuyao (EX-HN 4) and Sizhukong (SJ 23) as the starting points. This massage movement is performed in a type of criss-cross motion. The right thumb starts at the left eyebrow and wipes backwards and down towards the

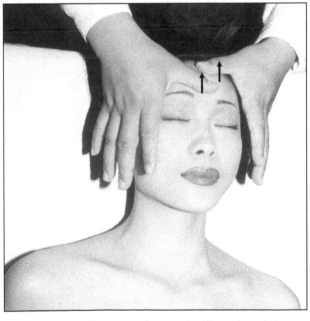

apex of the head. The left thumb starts at the right eyebrow and wipes backward and downward towards the apex of the head. Repeat this procedure 4-6 times.

Movement 3. Wiping the Forehead

Starting from the medial line, wipe from Yintang (EX-HN 3) in the center of the forehead laterally toward the hairline and to Taiyang (EX-HN 5) respectively. Repeat this procedure 4-6 times.

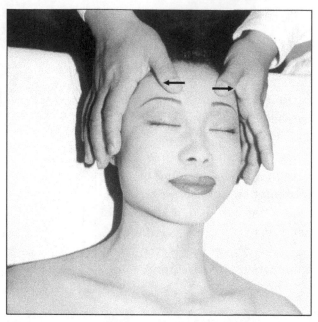

Movement 4. Kneading and Pressing Yuyao (EX-HN 4)

Using the pads of the middle fingers, knead and press Yuyao (EX-HN 4), the mid point of the eyebrows, 4-6 times. You can also begin this massage movement by pressing and kneading the medial end of the eyebrows 4-6 times

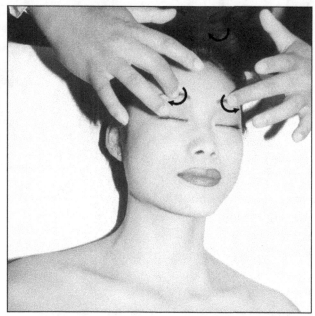

Movement 5. Kneading and Pressing Sizhukong (SJ 23)

Using the pads of both middle fingers, press and knead Sizhukong (SJ 23) in a circular motion 4-6 times.

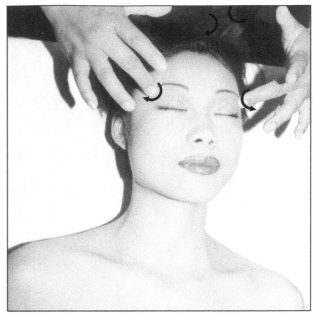

Movement 6. Scraping the Eyebrows

With the pads of both thumbs, start from Zanzhu (UB 2) and scrape along the eyebrow bone laterally to Sizhukong (SJ 23). Repeat this procedure 4-6 times

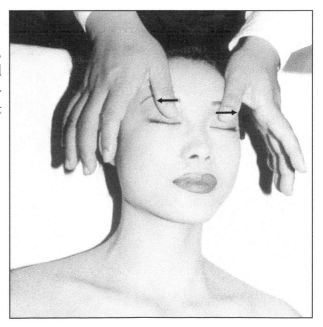

Movement 7. Wiping the Eyeball

During this manipulation, make sure the patient's eyes are closed. Using the pads of both thumbs, softly wipe laterally from Jingming (UB 1) to Tongziliao (GB 1). Repeat 4-6 times. You can begin by first wiping along the upper occipital bone, then across the closed eyeball, and finally along the lower occipital (eye socket)

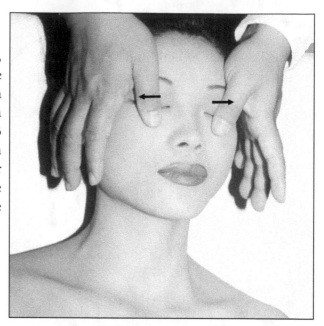

Movement 8. Kneading and Pressing Yingxiang (LI 20)

Place the pads of the thumbs or middle fingers on Yingxiang (LI 20), knead and press this point in circular motions until the patient feels a slight soreness. Repeat the procedure for 4 to 6 times. You can also begin this procedure by starting with circular kneading and pressing just below the inner canthuses of both eyes, down along the sides of the nose until you reach Yingxiang (LI 20), at the sides of the nostrils. Sequence movements Movement 8 through Movement 10 can all be performed in a continuous motion,

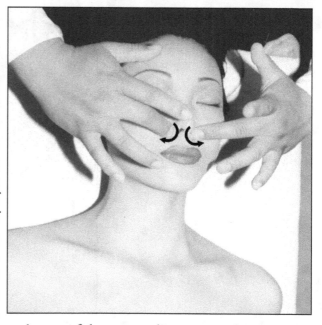

starting with pressing and kneading at the top of the nose and pausing at the important areas, such as Yingxiang (LI 20), then kneading and pressing along the specific path outlined in each manipulation. Remember to pause and press, and then knead with more strength at the points emphasized in the manipulation.

Movement 9. Kneading and Pressing Dicang (ST 4)

Place the pads of the middle fingers on Dicang (ST 4), which is at the corners of the mouth, and knead and press for about 4 to 6 times.

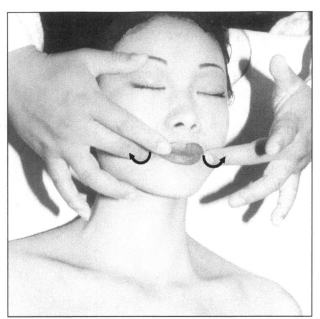

Movement 10. Pressing Specific Acupressure Points

Using the whorled pads of the middle fingers, knead and press successively from Daying (ST 5), Jiache (ST 6), Xiaguan (ST 7), Tinghui (GB 2), Tinggong (SI 19), Ermen (SJ 21) pressing only Shuaigu (GB 8) and Baihui (GV (Du) 20). Repeat the procedure for 4 to 6 times, in the order proposed.

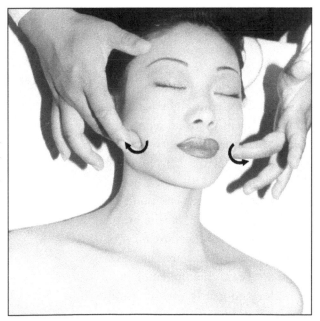

Movement 11. Kneading and Pressing Chengjiang (CV (Ren) 24)

Rest the pads of the thumb on Chengjiang (CV (Ren) 24), and middle finger of the right hand on Lianquan (CV (Ren) 23). Press and knead in a circular motion for about 4 to 6 times. Use the index and ring finger to support the middle finger, under the chin.

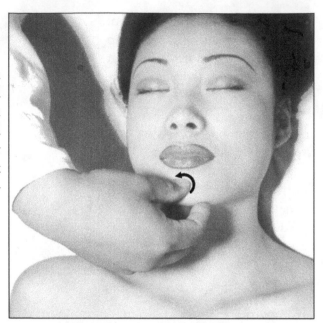

Movement 12. Stroking the Right Side of the Neck

Ask the patient to gently turn his or her head to the left side. Support the cheek with your left hand. Resting your right hand on the neck, gently stroke along the points Lianquan (CV (Ren) 23), Tiantu (CV (Ren) 22), Renying (ST 9), Futu (LI 18), and Quepen (ST 12). These points are found on the curved contour of the neck. Repeat the same procedure for 4 to 6 times. Because this area houses a major artery this manipulation is to be performed gently and smoothly from the middle of the neck to the side and towards the back of the head.

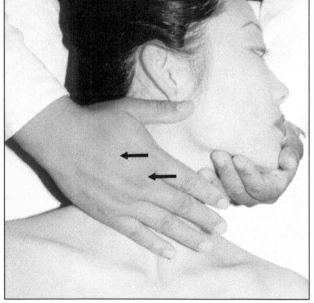

Movement 13. Scalp Sweeping Method (Right Side of Head)

You will be using the flat part and pads of the fingers, and the thumb as an alignment point for the other fingers. Place the thumb at the mid-point of the anterior hairline. Starting with the little finger, sweep each finger in succession like a wave, from the hairline at the corner of the forehead to the posterior ear and the posterior hairline, about 4 to 6 times. While performing this manipulation with the four fingers, the thumb simultaneously drags down the head toward the Baihui (GV (Du) 20), the apex of the head.

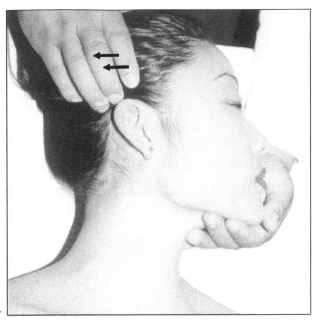

Movement 14. Scalp Finger-Combing Method (Right Side)

Continuing from the last massage movement, make claw-like fingers and begin to comb along the curve of the head from the anterior hairline all the way to the posterior hairline. Both hands should move/comb from the middle of the head to the posterior of the head. This motion moves along the bladder and gallbladder meridians. Repeat the same procedure 4 to 6 times.

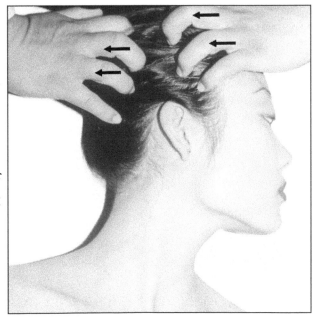

Movement 15. Massaging the Motor and Sensory Areas (Right Side)

With a gently closed hand, knead with the flat of the thumb from the apex of the head all the way to end of the lateral hairline in front of the ear. (This motion is sometimes referred to as the "Pac Man" motion, because of the way the hand inches its way across the head). Repeat the same procedure 4 to 6 times.

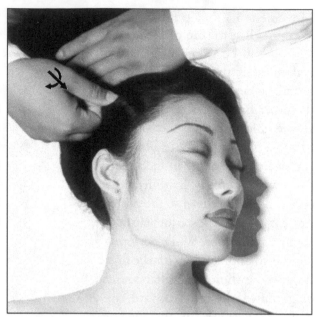

Movement 16. Finger Flicking Motor and Sensory Areas (Right Side)

Use the index or middle finger to flick slowly and softly on the right motor and sensory areas found along the lateral side of the head. Gently flick 2 to 4 times.

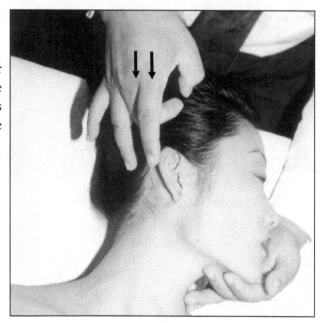

Movement 17. Kneading and Pressing the Auricular Helix (Right Side)

With the back of the right ear supported by the forefinger, middle, ring and little finger, and the flat of the thumb pressing the front side of the ear, softly and slowly move the thumb, kneading and pressing along the helix of the ear from top to bottom. The whorled surfaces/pads of the other fingers should be supporting the thumb as it descends along the ear. Repeat the same procedure 4 to 6 times.

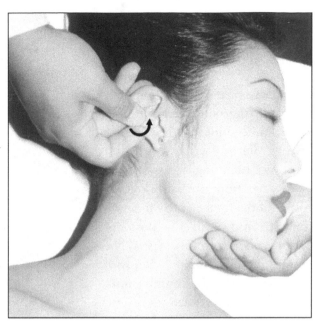

Movement 18. Stroking the Left Side of the Neck

Ask the patient to turn their head to the right side, supporting the cheek with your right hand. Resting the left hand on the neck, gently stroke the points Lianquan (CV (Ren) 23), Tiantu (CV (Ren) 22), Renying (ST 9), Futu (LI 18) and Quepen (ST 12) which are situated along the curved contour of the neck. Repeat the same procedure 4 to 6 times. Again, remember to apply only light and smooth pressure along the neck.

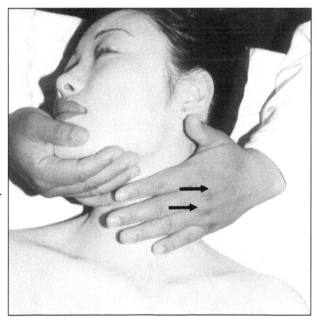

Movement 19. Scalp Sweeping Method (Left Side)

You will be using the flat part and pads of the fingers, and the thumb as an alignment point for the other fingers. Place the thumb at the mid-point of the anterior hairline. Starting with the little finger, sweep each finger in succession like a wave, from the hairline at the corner of the forehead to the posterior ear, and until the posterior hairline, about 4 to 6 times. While performing this manipulation with the four fingers, the thumb simultaneously drags down the head toward the Baihui (GV (Du) 20), the apex of the head.

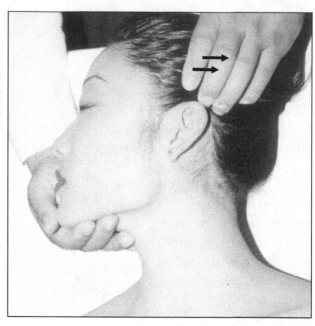

Movement 20. Scalp Finger-Combing Method (Left Side)

Continuing from the last massage movement, make claw-like fingers and begins to comb along the curve of the head from the anterior hairline all the way to the posterior hairline. Both hands should move/comb from the middle of the head to the posterior of the head. This motion moves along the bladder and gallbladder meridians. Repeat the same procedure 4 to 6 times.

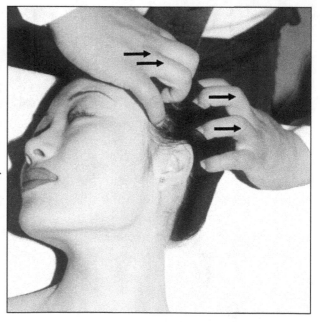

Movement 21. Massaging the Motor and Sensory Areas (Left Side)

With a gently closed hand, knead with the flat of the thumb from the apex of the head all the way to end of the lateral hairline in front of the ear using the "Pac Man" motion. Repeat the same procedure 4 to 6 times.

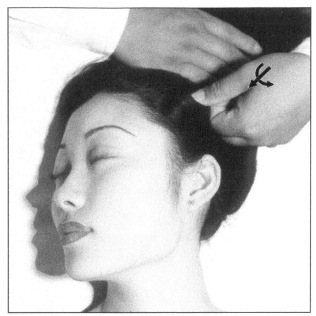

Movement 22. Finger Flicking Motor and Sensory Areas (Left Side)

Use the index or middle finger to flick slowly and softly on the left motor and sensory areas found along the lateral side of the head. Gently flick 2 to 4 times.

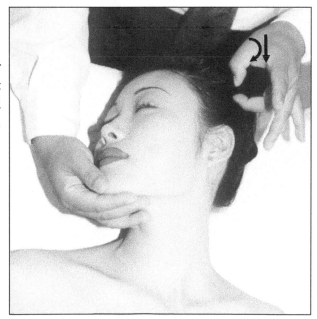

Movement 23. Kneading and Pressing the Auricular Helix (Left side)

With the back of the right ear supported by the forefinger, middle, ring, little finger, and the flat of the thumb pressing the front side of the ear, softly and slowly move the thumb, kneading and pressing along the helix of the ear from top to bottom. The whorled surfaces/pads of the other fingers should be supporting the thumb as it descends along the ear. Repeat the same procedure 4 to 6 times.

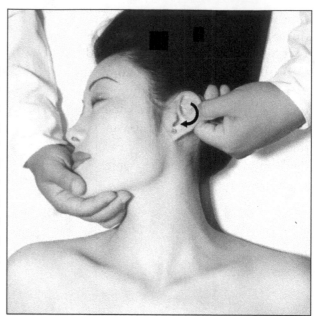

Movement 24. Stroking the Chin (Both Sides)

Place the index finger at Chengjiang (CV (Ren) 24), just under the lower lip. With the fingers encircling the lower jaw and chin, stroke the chin on both sides backwards toward Daying (ST 5) and the ear lobes. The thumbs should be raised and not touching the face during this manipulation. Repeat the same procedure 4 to 6 times.

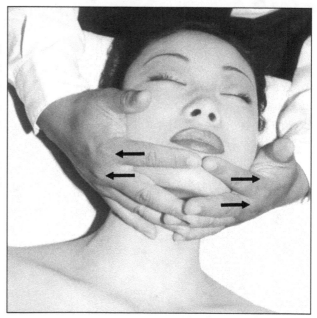

Movement 25. Stroking Shuigou (GV (Du) 26) (Both Sides of the Philtrum)

Continuing from the last massage movement, rest the index fingers on the philtrum, the groove just above the upper lip, and the middle fingers on the points of Chengjiang (CV (Ren) 24), just below the lower lip. With the chin encircled by the ring fingers and the little fingers, stroke the philtrum and Quanliao (SI 18) on both sides downwards toward Daying (ST 5) and the ear lobes, 4 to 6 times.

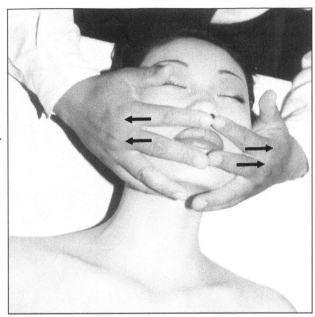

Movement 26. Stroking Jingming (UB 1) Downwards and Raising the Chin Upwards

Rest the pads of both thumbs on the points of Jingming (UB 1), which is near the inner canthuses, just at the beginning of the bridge of the nose. Stroke along both sides of the nose downwards to Yingxiang (LI 20) and Dicang (ST 4), the corner of the lips. Simultaneously, with the chin encircled by the other fingers, raise the muscle of the chin upwards slowly and softly 4 to 6 times.

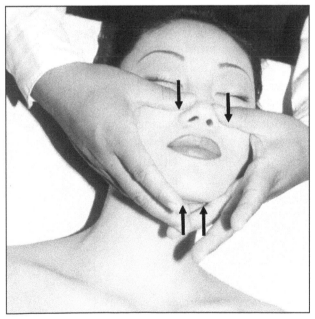

Movement 27. Downward Squeezing of the Nose

While supporting the lower chin with the left hand, place the right index and middle fingers over the nose and gently squeeze and sweep downward along the points from Jingming (UB 1) to Yingxiang (LI 20). Repeat the same procedure 4 to 6 times.

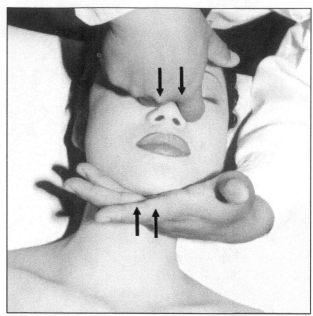

Movement 28. Kneading the Temple—Taiyang (EX-HN 5)

Place both thumbs on the forehead at the mid-point of the anterior hairline. Then make a lightly cupped fist, while slightly bending the index finger and placing it on the temples. Knead the temples, Taiyang (EX-HN 5) with the outside side of the index finger. Repeat 4 to 6 times.

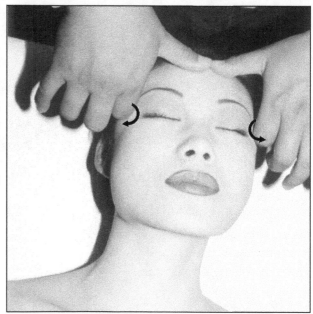

Movement 29. Circular Rubbing of the Face

In this massage movement, the practitioner's hands are also placed at opposite corners of the patient's face. For instance, when the practitioner's right hand is wiping across the left side of the chin, the left hand should be wiping across the right corner of the forehead. With the palms of both hands, trace along the sides of the face from the mandible all the way up to the forehead, rubbing/wiping alternately 4 to 6 times.

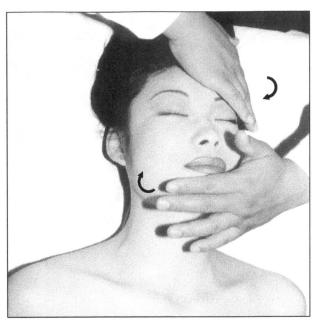

Movement 30. Digital Pressing Fengchi (GB 20)

Place the flats or pads of the middle fingers tightly on the Fengchi (GB 20), and press it in circular motions 4 to 6 times. You can also press, and then gently but firmly pull backwards on this point.

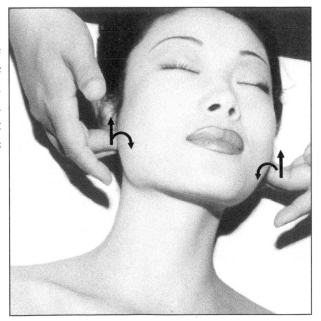

Movement 31. Digital Pressing Yifeng (SJ 17)

This manipulation is the same as 30, but this time you place the pads of the middle fingers tightly on Yifeng (SJ 17) (back of earlobes), and again press them 4 to 6 times.

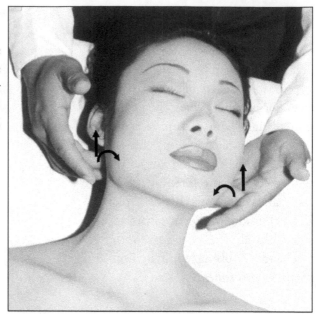

Movement 32. Digital Pressing Baihui (GV (Du) 20)

Now place the pads of both thumbs strongly on Baihui (GV (Du) 20), and press it about 4 to 6 times. You can press this point strongly, but make sure to confirm how strong with the patient.

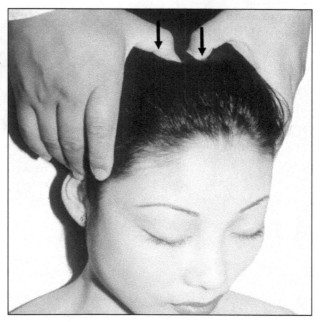

Movement 33. Digital Pressing Sishencong (EX-HN 1)

Put the flats of the thumbs tightly on the Sishencong (EX-HN 1), pressing for about 4 to 6 times. The area you stimulate is above and below, and on both sides of Baihui (GV (Du) 20).

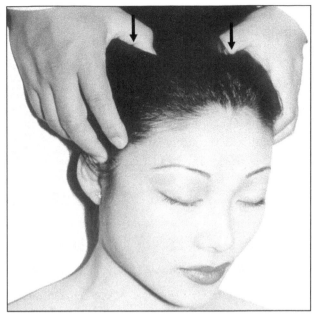

Movement 34. Thenar Rolling of the Forehead

With the minor thenar eminence and the ulna dorsum of the hand (meaty part at side and below the little finger), apply a rolling and kneading pressure along the surface of the forehead. Roll and knead the forehead for about 4 to 6 times.

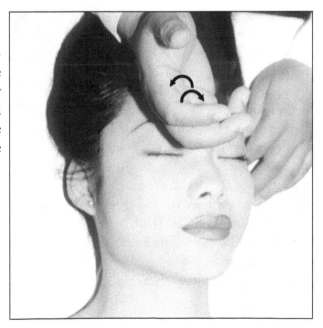

Movement 35. Pressing and Wiping the Forehead with the Root of the Palm

Using the bottom of the palm, slowly and softly press and wipe the forehead, starting from the middle, toward the apex of the head. Use both hands alternately to cover both sides of the forehead. Repeat 4 to 6 times.

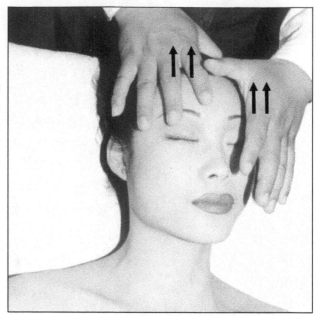

Movement 36. Fingers Combing and Wiping the Forehead

This manipulation is similar to the previous one, except this time you apply pressure with the fingers instead of the palm root only. Exerting pressure with the flats of the fingers on the forehead, slowly and softly comb and wipe the forehead with both hands, alternately, in a straight line from Yintang (EX-HN 3) to Shenting (GV (Du) 24), Shangxing (GV (Du) 23), Zanzhu (UB 2), Quchai (UB 4), Yuyao (EX-HN 4), Toulinqi (GB 15), Sizhukong (SJ 23), Touwei (ST 8), to the top of the head, 4 to 6 times.

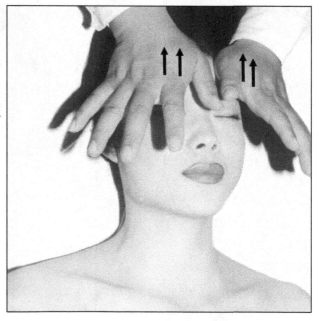

Movement 37. Qi Stroking of the Face

Continuing from the last massage movement, gradually remove the hands from the head. Stroke slowly and softly over the face concentrating on the Qi of the hands. This is a form of energy massage where no physical contact with the body surface is necessary. Repeat 4 to 6 times.

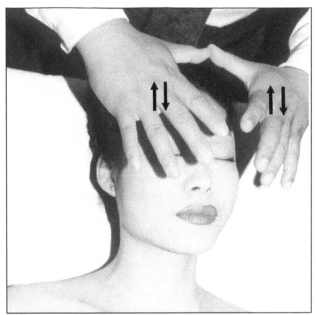

Movement 38. Finger Flicking the Forehead

Flick the index or middle finger on the forehead across the entire surface of the forehead slowly and softly, 2 to 4 times. (Similar to Movement 16 and Movement 22)

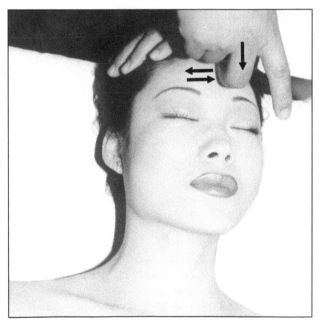

Movement 39. Forehead Tapping with Clasped/Cupped Hands

Gently clasp/cup the hands together; slightly flex the joints so that the palms form a hollow palmar cup. Tap the forehead with the back of the hand for about 4 to 6 times.

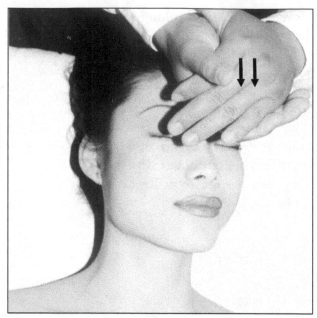

Movement 40. Forehead Tapping with Hollow Fists

With hollow fists, tap slowly and softly on the forehead with the radial side of the little fingers, from the middle of the forehead to both sides. You can perform this tapping in circular motions, covering the entire surface of the forehead. Repeat 4 to 6 times.

Manipulation 40 is the last one performed while the patient is in a supine position.

The following massage movements are performed while the patient is in a seated position. Use a firm chair instead of having the patient sit on a massage table.

Movement 41. Pressing and Squeezing Both Sides of the Head

Place both palms on the sides of the head of the patient, your palm roots should be positioned just above the ears. Slowly and softly, squeeze/press the head inwards 4 to 6 times. You should apply strong pressure, but not cause the patient any extreme discomfort.

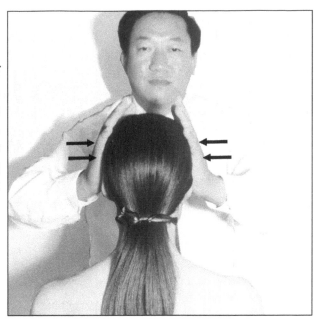

Movement 42. Ming Tiangu (also referred to as Inner Ear Vibration)

The practitioner places both palms on the ears of the patient, with the hearts of the palms pointing to the front and the fingers to the back of the head. Use the palm root to fold the ear over (toward the front). Place the index finger on top of the middle finger, and flick the protruding bone (occipital bone) behind the ears 10 times. This will produce a booming/vibrating sound in the ears. Instead of the usual way that sounds vibrate through the ear canal (externally to

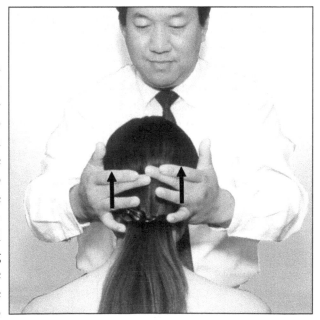

internally), this manipulation produces internal stimulation of the ear.

Movement 43. Lifting and Scrubbing the Head

Place both hands on the head as if holding a ball, then lift and scrub swiftly and repeatedly 4 to 6 times. Start at the top of the head and then repeat the same manipulation to the middle, back, and lower parts of the head.

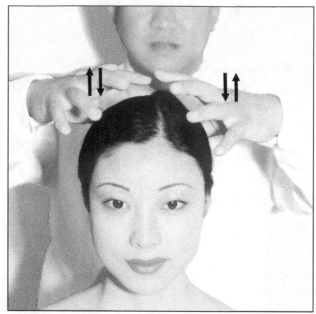

Movement 44. Finger Tapping the Head

Place both hands on the head as if holding a ball, and then swiftly and gently tap using the fingers, from the apex of head down to the shoulder. Repeat 4 to 6 times.

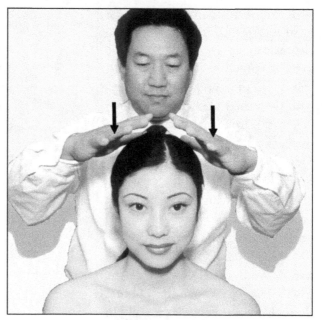

Movement 45. Kneading and Grasping the Neck Tendons

To support the patient's head, place the left hand on the forehead. Hold the tendons and muscle bundles of the neck with the thumb, index, and middle finger symmetrically. Knead and grasp them, in an up-down manipulation. Repeat 4 to 6 times.

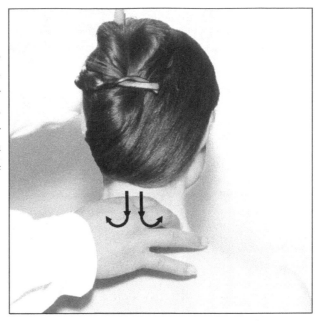

Movement 46. Rubbing and Sweeping the Posterior Hairline

Using the backs (inner portions) of the thumb, index, and middle fingers together, lift and sweep the skin of the posterior hairline and neck downwards toward the back. When beginning this manipulation, rub the points on the sides and middle of the neck softly. Repeat 4 to 6 times.

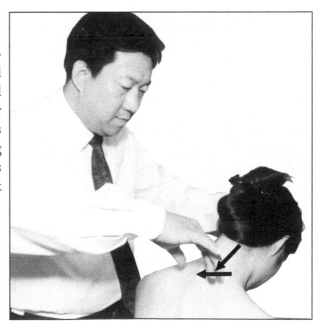

Movement 47. Pushing and Pressing the Sternocleido-mastoid Muscle

For this manipulation, the practitioner should stand behind and slightly to the left side of the patient. With the patient's head inclined to the left side, using the left hand slightly raise the head while supporting the chin with the hand. Open the thumb of the right hand at a 90-degree angle. Rest the whorled surface/pad of the thumb on the top of the sternocleidomastoid muscle. Then press and push the thumb slowly and softly along the muscle from the top to the bot-

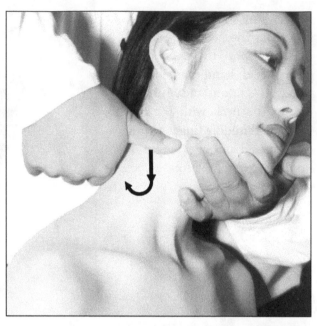

tom of the neck to the sternocleid joint. Repeat 4 to 6 times. Repeat this manipulation on the right side of the patient's neck.

Movement 48. Squeezing the Neck

Ask the patient to bend/lower their head to their chest. Standing behind the patient, the practitioner clasps both hands and with the palms facing inward and conforms the hands to the shape of the neck. Then squeeze the neck by pushing inwards and lifting the palm roots in a squeeze-and-relax alternation. Repeat 4 to 6 times.

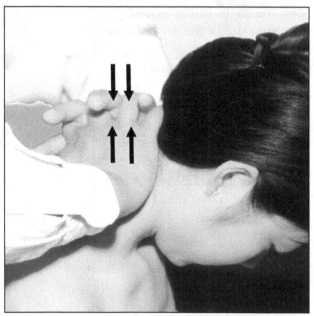

Movement 49. Kneading and Pressing Dazhui (GV (Du) 14)

Rest the whorled surfaces/pads of both thumbs on Dazhui (GV (Du) 14) (cervical vertebrae 7). Knead and press in a circular motion 4 to 6 times.

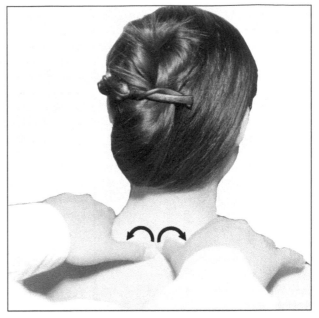

Movement 50. Rolling and Pressing the Neck

Standing behind the patient, the practitioner rests the minor thenar eminence of both hands on the end of the neck and beginning of the shoulders, with the hands and fingers slightly bent and in a relaxed position. From the mid-point of the shoulders (Dazhui GV (Du) 14), roll and press the shoulders laterally toward the outer joints of the shoulder. Repeat 4 to 6 times.

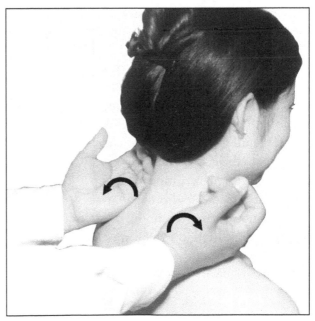

Movement 51. Grasping and Lifting the Shoulders

Hold the tendons and muscle bundles of the shoulders with the thumbs and another finger symmetrically (using either the index or middle fingers). Rhythmically grasp and lift the tendons and muscles in a squeeze-and-relax rotation from the center of the shoulders to the sides. Repeat 4 to 6 times.

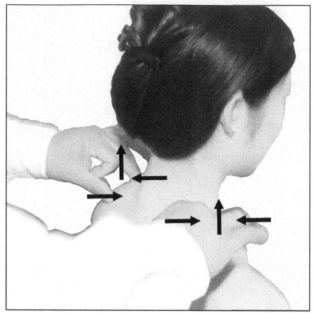

Movement 52. Tapping the Neck and Shoulders with Hollow Fists

Form a hollow fist. Tap the neck and shoulder areas from the left to right side. When tapping, the little fingers make contact with the neck and shoulder regions, and the other fingers naturally press against each other creating a snapping sound. You can also use a circular motion when performing this manipulation. Repeat 4 to 6 times.

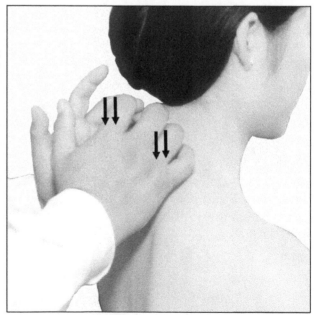

Movement 53. Tapping Neck and Shoulder with Clasped/Cupped Hands

Place the two hands in a clapping or clasped fashion, with the joints of the hands slightly flexed in order to create a space between the palms (creating a cupped effect). Use the back of the hand to tap the neck and shoulder regions from left to right. Repeat 4 to 6 times.

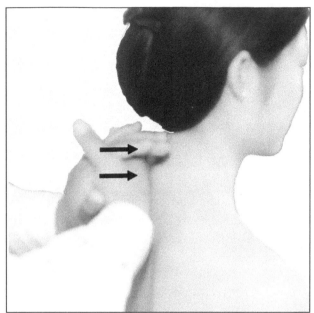

Movement 54. Patting the Neck and Shoulders with Concave Palm

Close the fingers of one hand (line them together), and slightly flex the joints in order to concave the palm (make a cupped palm). Pat on the neck and shoulders with the concave palm from the left to right side of the neck, shoulders, and upper back. Repeat 4 to 6 times.

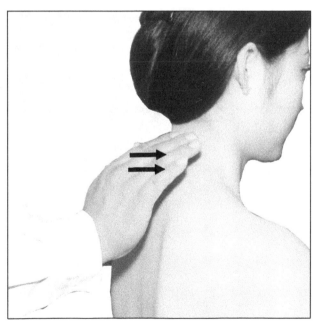

Movement 55. Spreading the Chest

Ask the patient to cross their fingers behind their head, opening up the arms and spreading the elbows. The practitioner stands behind the patient and places the palms of his hands against the patient's elbows, drawing them back to spread the chest open. The practitioner's right knee should be raised against the thoracic vertebrae (middle region) of the patient's back for this procedure. Repeat 4 to 6 times.

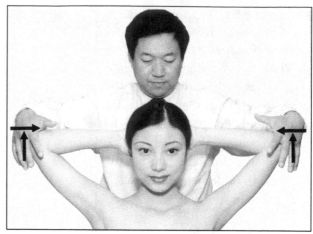

Movement 56. Rotating the Shoulders

Remaining in the same position, and continuing from the last massage movement, the practitioner now begins to rotate the arms by moving the elbows with his palms in an up, down, front, and back rotational motion. Repeat this procedure 2 to 4 times.

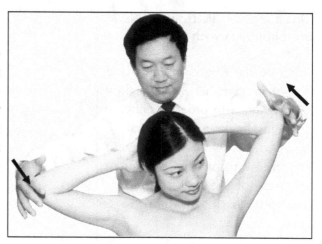

Movement 57. Forearm Tapping with Cupped Fist

Standing at the side of the patient, support the patient's outstretched arm by holding the wrist with your left hand. Make a hollow fist with the right hand. Start from the wrist, tapping up along the inner, middle, and outer aspects of the arm respectively. Tap each side of the arm 4 to 6 times. Repeat this procedure with both arms.

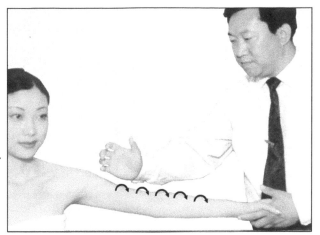

Movement 58. Wiping the Back of the Hand

The practitioner holds the patient's hand in between both of his hands. Place the thumbs on the back of the hand and press the other fingers against the palm. With the flat of the thumbs tightly adhering to the back of the patient's hand, wipe the thumb from the center towards the sides of the hand. Repeat the procedure 4 to 6 times on each hand.

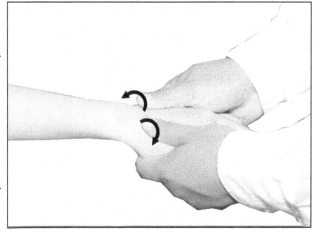

Movement 59. Holding-Twisting the Fingers

Hold the patients arms at the wrist. Hold one finger between the thumb and the index finger. Knead and twist all the way from the root of the finger to the tip. Repeat the procedure 2 to 4 times for each finger on both hands.

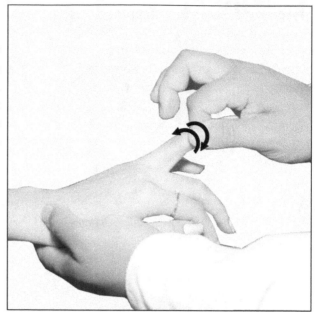

Movement 60. Traction of the Finger Joints

Hold the patient's wrist with one hand. Hold the root of the finger between the flexed (bent) middle and index fingers. Smooth/sweep downwards with a quick pulling motion, from the root to the tip of the finger. At the tip of the finger, pull slightly harder and quickly and this should create a snapping sound. Repeat the procedure 2 to 4 times for each finger on each hand.

You have now completed a full Wu's Head Massage treatment sequence.

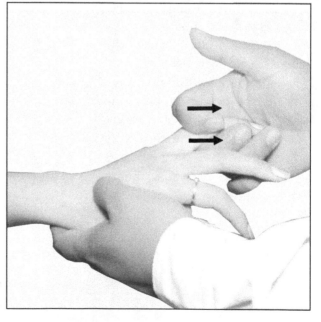

CHAPTER 10

Health and Cosmetic Effects of Wu's Head Massage

Eventually, we will all have to face the innumerable changes that our bodies will experience as a result of growing older. Because it is our face that greets others on a daily basis, the most noticeable change is usually the emergence of wrinkles on the forehead, corners of the eyes, and then the eventual softening and weakening of the rest of the body. With the onset of wrinkles, the skin slowly develops a saggy and dry appearance, sometimes with maculae (age spots) sprinkled across the skin's surface. Almost simultaneously, the hair begins to grow thinner, and eventually turns grey. Like withered autumn leaves, hairs begin to fall from the head.

The eventual slowing down of our cellular metabolism results in the very apparent aging process. For example, the glands (known as sebaceous glands) underneath the skin undergo atrophy, the subcutaneous fat deposits decline, the pigments condense, and the list of changes goes on. The underlying causes for aging is also related to the state of the internal organs. Assuming that the internal organs are functioning well, simple treatments to care for the skin can act as a natural preventive measure of the common visual aging effects, and can account for a healthier appearance.

Massage enhances blood circulation, thereby promoting cell regeneration and increasing cell elasticity. Cells are then more capable of absorbing nutrients, and the skin becomes smoother and softer.

Anti-Aging Massage Treatments

Treatment for Wrinkles and Facial Aging

To prevent and inhibit wrinkles from emerging on the face, we perform the following massage movements from the Wu's Head Massage Sequence:

Movement 1. Kneading and Pressing Zanzhu (UB 2)

Movement 2. Wiping Forehead Meridians (Alternately)

Movement 3. Wiping the Forehead

Movement 34. Thenar Rolling of the Forehead

Movement 35. Pressing and Wiping the Forehead with the Root of the Palm

Movement 38. Finger Flicking the Forehead

Movement 36. Fingers Combing and Wiping the Forehead

Movement 39. Forehead Tapping with Clasped/Cupped Hands

Movement 40. Tapping the Forehead with Hollow Fists

Function. These massage movements help to smooth out the wrinkles, and work as an effective prevention for headaches, forehead ache, dizziness, and insomnia.

Treatment for Eye Ailments Caused by Aging

During the aging process, many other side effects occur that are more detrimental than the aesthetic affects, such as aging. Blurred vision and "eye bags" are commonly seen in aging adults.

To address these problems, we perform the following massage movements of the WHM sequence:

Movement 6. Scraping the Eyebrows

Movement 7. Wiping the Eyeball

Movement 26. Stroking Jingming (UB 1) Downwards and Raising the Chin Upwards

Movement 28. Kneading the Temple—Taiyang (EX-HN 5)

Movement 1. Kneading and Pressing Zanzhu (UB 2)

Movement 4. Kneading and Pressing Yuyao (EX-HN 4)

Movement 5. Kneading and Pressing Sizhukong (SJ 23)

Function. These massage movements aid in smoothing out wrinkles around the eye, improving vision, and preventing bags under the eyes. These massage movements are also effective in the prevention of headaches, pain in the eye-socket, migraine, insomnia, blurred vision, myopia and glaucoma.

Treatment for Nose Ailments Caused by Aging

To address the need to increase circulation of the nose area, we perform the following massage movements

Movement 8. Kneading and Pressing Yingxiang (LI 20)

Movement 26. Stroking Jingming (UB 1) Downwards and Raising the Chin Upwards

Movement 27. Downward Squeezing of the Nose

Function. These manipulations promote circulation so they are able to prevent rhinocleisis, allergic rhinitis, chronic rhinitis, and paranasal sinusitis.

Treatments for Stress-Related Ailments

We have all, at some point, in our lives, been overwhelmed by our busy lifestyles, demands from work, modern society, family, and unhealthy dietary habits. All of these, over the years, have caused us to experience increasingly higher rates of stress and stress-related health problems. This has undoubtedly contributed to an early onset of the aging process and the appearance of aging.

To relax the facial muscles, and improve local circulation, we use the following massage movements:

Movement 10. Pressing Specific Acupressure Points

Movement 24. Stroking the Chin (Both Sides)

Movement 25. Stroking Shuigou (GV (Du) 26) (Both Sides of the Philtrum)

Movement 26. Stroking Jingming (UB 1) Downwards and Raising the Chin Upwards

Movement 55. Spreading the Chest

Movement 56. Rotating the Shoulders

Importance of Touch

Humans and most species not only enjoy, but also need physical contact; they need to be touched. This is an innate quality that is necessary for growth, whether emotionally, intellectually or physically. Children demonstrate this natural tendency toward affection and physical contact more directly than adults do (most likely a result of our individualistic and fast-paced environments created by society).

Treatments for Relaxation and Rejuvenation

The following massage movements create a most necessary role in inducing a sedative and hypnotic-like state that enables the body to restore energy quickly, soothes and calms the mind, and encourages a natural and consistent circulation.

Movement 1. Kneading and Pressing Zanzhu (UB 2)

Movement 7. Wiping the Eyeball

Movement 12 and Movement 18. Stroking the Right and Left Sides of the Neck

Function. The thin, small part of the carotid sinus artery lies in the upper portion of the neck. The nerve endings of this artery serve as pressure receptors or baroreceptors, and are highly sensitive to changes in blood pressure within the artery. Softly massaging this area can adjust the heart rate and normalize the blood pressure. Similar effects can also be found by gently massaging the closed eyeball. Massage Movement 7 (Wiping the Eyeball), and Movement 12 and Movement 18 (Stroking the Right and Left Sides of the Neck) aim for this result. In addition, these methods are effective for the prevention of laryngitis, tonsillitis, thyroid enlargement, headache, insomnia, and menopause syndrome.

Effects of Ear Manipulations

As we have outlined earlier in this book (see page 56), the distribution of auricular points is similar to an inverted fetus inside. Different points govern different regions of the body, including the facial area. Anti-aging, although usually a concern for those worried about aesthetic changes, more importantly has a direct link to the well being of the internal organs.

Through the network of the meridians and collaterals, the state of internal organs is reflected in the color of the face. For example, liver and kidney-based diseases create a dark green complexion, while gastro-internal related diseases result in a yellowish complexion. Whenever the functions of the internal organs are thwarted, the face becomes sallow.

Treatments for Stimulating Internal Organs

Since the ear is seen as a blueprint/microcosm of the body, to assist with internal functions causing aging, we can massage using the following massage movements:

Movement 17 and Movement 23. Kneading and Pressing the Right and Left Auricular Helices

FUNCTIONS

These massage movements stimulate the internal organs, which in turn, prevents many of the causes of aging. These treatments are also an effective way to prevent ear infections, tinnitus, and declining hearing.

Encouraging Hair Growth

It is common knowledge that as we age, our hair grows thinner, turns white and eventually falls off.

Treatments for Hair Growth

The following massage movements are used to delay this transition:

Movement 13 and Movement 19. Sweeping of the Right and Left Scalp

Movement 14 and Movement 20. Finger Combing the Scalp (Both Sides)

Movement 15 and Movement 21. Massaging the Motor and Sensory Area (Both Sides)

Movement 16 and Movement 22. Flicking the Motor and Sensory Areas (Both Sides)

Movement 30. Digital Pressing Fengchi (GB 20)

Movement 31. Digital Pressing Yifeng (SJ 17)

Movement 32. Digital Pressing Baihui (GV (Du) 20)

Movement 33. Digital Pressing Sishencong (EX-HN 1)

Movement 41. Pressing and Squeezing Both Sides of the Head

Movement 43. Lifting and Scrubbing

Movement 44. Finger Tapping the Head

Function. By massaging the head, we increase local blood circulation. Hair growth depends on blood circulation. These massage movements are also effective for treating headaches, dizziness, forgetfulness, and neurasthenia.

Wai Qi

Wai Qi is the act of emitting Qi or energy to improve the health of a patient. Wai Qi is used in many styles of massage. Its effects are far-reaching—from having a more sedative and calming effect, to treating diseases and pains, and to increasing circulation. Although a skilled and experienced practitioner would use Qi when performing the entire massage, there are some movements that stress the importance of emitting Qi, more than others. In these sequences, the practitioner is using his or her Qi to encourage the patient's Qi to flow easily and gently throughout the body. The skill of emitting Qi is developed through Qigong practice (see Chapter 12)

Movements Using Wai Qi

Movement 37. Qi Stroking of the Face

Function. This massage movement increases local blood circulation. It also invigorates the brain, improves intelligence, and has cosmetic enhancement effects. It is also effective in the treatment of headaches, dizziness, insomnia, amnesia, and neurosis.

Releasing Tension in the Neck

As one ages a number of mobility problems ensue, and these are frequently reflected in the neck area. The bones age and the once-flexible vertebrae calcify. Stiff necks effect the very crucial massage movements of the head.

Treatments for Healing the Neck

The following massage movements focus on decreasing and preventing problems with the neck:

Movement 49. Kneading and Pressing Dazhui (GV (Du) 14)
Movement 46. Rubbing and Sweeping the Posterior Hairline
Movement 45. Kneading and Grasping the Neck Tendons
Movement 47. Pushing and Pressing the Sternocleidomastoid Muscle
Movement 48. Squeezing the Neck
Movement 50. Rolling and Pressing the Neck
Movement 51. Grasping and Lifting the Shoulders
Movement 52. Tapping the Neck and Shoulders with Hollow Fists
Movement 53. Tapping Neck and Shoulder with Clasped/Cupped Hands
Movement 54. Patting the Neck and Shoulders with Concave Palm

Function. These massage movements enhance the circulation in the head and neck areas, thus correcting the displacement of the vertebra and preventing neck-related problems. These massage movements are also effective for headaches, insomnia, and stiffened necks.

Finger Massage

There are three Yang meridians that directly connect the hands to the head and facial regions. There are three Yin meridians that connect with the hands' Yang meridians, via the acupuncture points on the fingertips. This connection allows the Yin meridians to indirectly connect with the head and facial regions.

Treatments for Massaging the Fingers

The following massage movements are used on the fingers:

Movement 57. Forearm Tapping with Cupped Fist

Movement 58. Wiping the Back of the Hand

Movement 59. Holding-Twisting the Fingers

Movement 60. Traction of the Finger Joints

Function. These massage movements are used to stimulate the meridian source (Jin-well points) at the fingertips. They not only serve as preventive measures for finger numbness and spasm, but also as a final step to quickly awaken the patient from the relaxed sedative state often induced during massage.

PART V
Practitioner's Self-Care

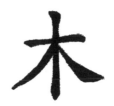

CHAPTER 11
Self-Care Treatments

Although this is the final chapter, it could easily have been the first. In the field of healing, self-maintenance should not be overlooked nor underrated. The simple truth is that when a person is healthy it is much easier to heal others.

Personal hygiene is an important area for anyone communicating with others. It is often a reflection of our mental and spiritual health. For the purposes of Wu's Head Massage, this means keeping the body clean and well groomed. The hands should be washed and the fingernails clean and trimmed short. Avoid overpowering perfume or cologne, as this may not agree with the patient.

Teaching health should be done by example. If you have habits that you feel are not good then this may be a good time to decrease or quit them altogether.

For a simple self-care program, we teach self-massage and Qigong. Self-massage of the head not only promotes personal health and appearance it is a very effective way of improving the skill of the Wu's Head Massage practitioner. Qigong is used to build the practitioner's energy and enable the practitioner to direct the body's energy from the core (Dantian) to the palms.

Some of these self-massage techniques are similar to the sixty massage movements described in Chapter 9.

Applying Simple Massage Techniques to Your Head and Face:

Self-Massage for the Eyes

1) Kneading Zanzhu (UB 2)

Apply the pads of the thumbs on Zanzhu (UB 2) in the depressions at the medial ends of the eyebrows. Knead this area with the thumbs 10 times. The force of kneading should be increased gradually until a slight feeling of soreness and distention occurs.

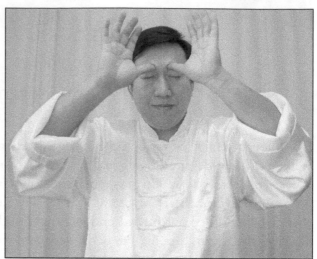

2) Kneading Jingming (UB 1)

Place the thumb and the index finger of the right hand on Jingming (UB 1) which is located in the depression, 0.1 cun above the inner canthus (inner corners of the eyes). Alternate between pressing downwards and pinching 10 times.

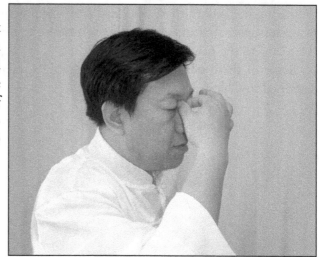

3) Pressing-Kneading Sibai (ST 2)

Place the index fingers on Sibai (ST 2) which is located 1 cun under the midpoint of the lower orbit (eye bone), and press-knead 10 times until you feel the sensation of slight soreness and distention.

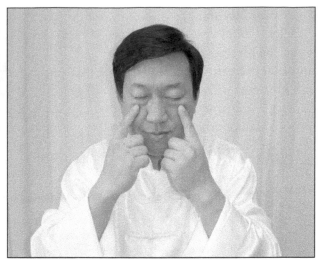

4) Scraping the Orbits

Bending the index fingers, apply their radial sides against the internal aspects of the upper orbits (upper eye bone) and scrape from the inner canthus to the outer. Continue the scraping with the lower orbits in the same way, for 10 times.

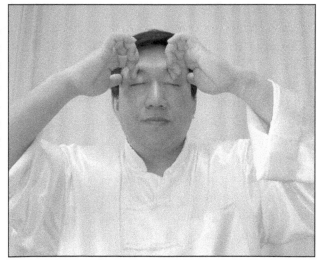

111

5) "Ironing" the Eyes

Close yours eyes slightly. Rub yours hands against each other until they create heat, and then cover the eyes with your palms as if "ironing" the eyes for about 30 seconds. Follow this procedure by rubbing the eyes gently 10 or more times.

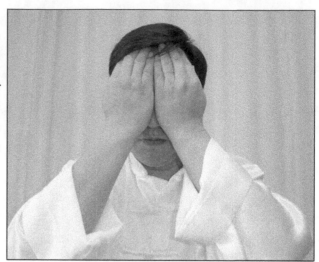

6) Kneading the Temple—Taiyang (EX-HN 5)

Apply strong pressure on Taiyang (EX-HN 5), with the pads of the thumbs or index fingers. Follow by kneading for 10 times until you feel a sensation of slight soreness and distention.

Function. These manipulations are effective for the prevention and treatment of myopia, blurred vision, glaucoma, optic atrophy, and other eye diseases.

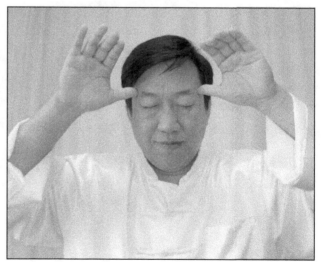

Self-Massage for the Nose

1) Pressing-Kneading Yingxiang (LI 20)

Rest the pads of the index fingers on Yingxiang (LI 20), then press and knead them 10 times or until you feel the sensation of soreness and distention.

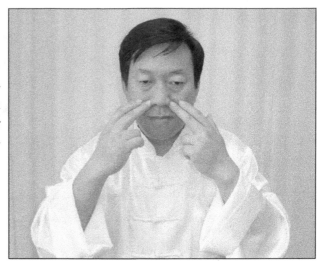

2) Rubbing the Nose (Sides)

Using the index or middle fingers of both hands, rub them against each other until you have created some heat. Then use these fingers to rub the nasolabial grooves (sides of the nostrils) up and down to warm them up. Repeat 10 times.

Function. These manipulations are effective for the prevention and treatment of colds, stuffy and running noses, allergic rhinitis, chronic rhinitis, and paranasal sinusitis.

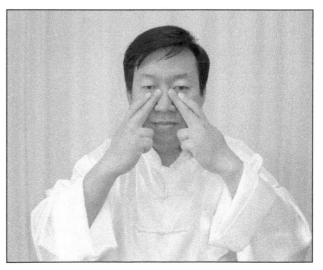

Self-massage for the Ears

1) Pressing-Kneading Points Surrounding the Ear

With the tips of the thumbs or the middle fingers, press and knead Ermen (SJ 21), Tinggong (SI 19), Tinghui (GB 2), and Yifeng (SJ 17) 10 times each or until you feel a sensation of soreness or distention.

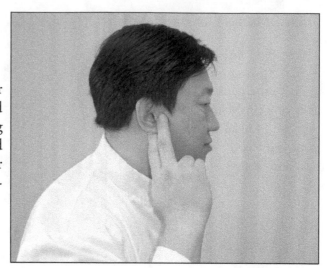

2) Rubbing the Helix of the Ear

Gently pinch the helices of the ear with the thumbs and the radial sides of the index fingers. Then rub upwards and downwards repeatedly 10 times or until the helices become hot.

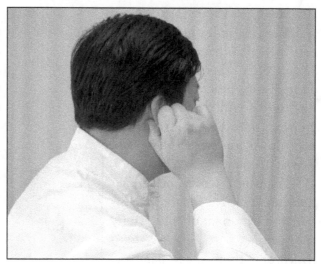

3) Ming Tiangu

Press both palms on the ears, with the root of the palms pointing forwards and the fingers pointing backwards. Place the index fingers on top of the middle fingers and flick the protruded bones (occipital bone) behind the ears 10 times. This will produce a booming sound in the ears. Most of the vibratory stimulation that our ears receive comes through the external ear and inwardly. This manipulation creates the vibration in the inner ear, outwardly.

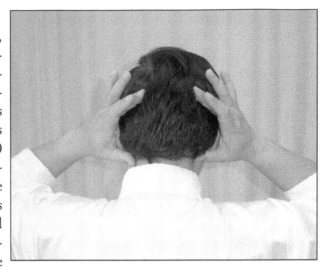

Function. These manipulations are effective for the prevention and treatment of tinnitus, deafness, and other ear problems

Self-massage for the Head

1) Forehead Pushing (Both sides of the head)

Bend the two index fingers and using the radial sides push along the midline of the forehead, which runs from Yintang (EX-HN 3) (also known as Third Eye) to the anterior hairline. Press outwards to the left and right sides of the head until you reach Taiyang (EX-HN 5) (also referred to as the temples), Sizhukong (SJ 23), and Touwei (ST 8). Repeat this sequence 10 times.

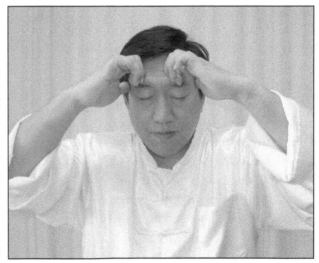

2) Wiping the Temples

Press the temples with the whorled surfaces/pads of the thumbs and proceed to wipe forcefully backwards. Repeat 10 times. This manipulation should produce a slight sensation of soreness and distention.

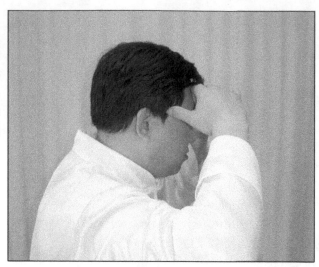

3) Pressing-Kneading Skull (Back of the Head)

Place the whorled surfaces/pads or tips of the thumbs firmly on Fengchi (GB 20) (the depressions below the occipital bone) and press them 10 or more times. Follow this manipulation with circular kneading. Continue by kneading the points of Naokong (GB 19) 10 times or until there is a sensation of slight soreness and distention.

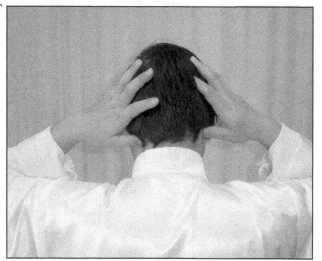

4) Pressing-Kneading Baihui (GV (Du) 20) and Sishencong (EX-HN 1)

Place the tips of the middle fingers on Baihui (GV (Du)) and press/knead 8-10 times. Do the same for Sishencong (EX-HN 1), the points beside, above and below Baihui (GV (Du) 20), 2-4 times.

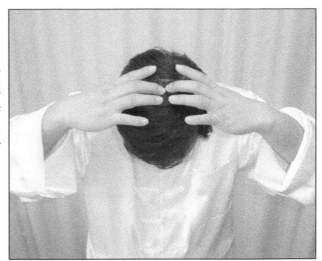

5) "Bathing the Face"

Rub the hands against each until they become warm. Place the palms lightly against the forehead, then rub firmly down to the mandibles (jawbone), along the mandible margins on the sides of the face towards Jiache (ST 6), and then upwards via the pre-auricular area (in front of the ears) toward the temples and end at the midpoint of the forehead. Repeat the sequence 6-8 times or until the face feels warm.

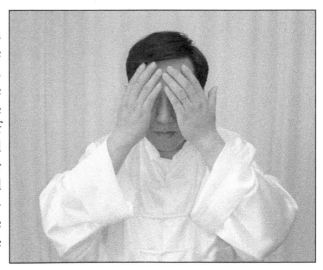

Function. These manipulations invigorate the brain, improve intelligence, and tranquilize the mind. They are effective in the treatment of headaches, dizziness, insomnia, amnesia, neurosis, and facial paralysis.

CHAPTER 12

Qigong for the Practitioner

Standing Qigong

Qigong is made up of two words: Qi is life energy (see page 5) and gong which means skill developed over time. Qigong is a type of Chinese exercise used to build and strengthen both the physical body and Qi of the practitioner.

Qigong is used to strengthen the energy of the practitioner. The Chinese say "Between heaven and earth is Man." This statement can be used to illustrate the basic posture of standing Qigong. There are three types of Qi—heaven Qi (Yang), earth Qi (Yin), and human Qi. According to TCM philosophy, a person can stand with mind and breathe on the heavens and legs firmly rooted in the earth, and thereby balance Yin and Yang energy in the body. The mind is allowed to go quiet, and peaceful nature-based images are drawn upon.

Breathing is natural and deepens into the lower abdominal area as Qi is allowed to sink within the body. Over time, the mind is trained to become quiet, relaxed, and focused, and the body naturally follows. The result of a daily energy exercise routine will result in a healthier practitioner, and this in turn will be passed onto the patient.

The two postures illustrated Three Circle Stance (Figure 12-1) and Embracing Post (Figure 12-2) should be practiced for about 15 minutes daily.

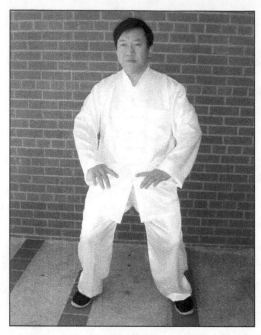

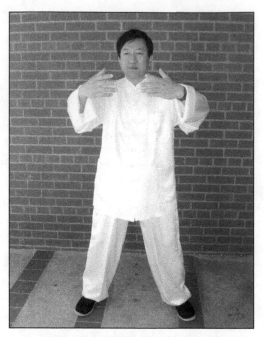

FIGURE 12-1 THREE CIRCLE STANCE POSTURE   FIGURE 12-2 EMBRACING POST POSTURE

Moving Qigong

The standing postures are the energy foundation of the practitioner. These static exercises are also the foundation of movement. The Moving Qigong that we practice is known as the 15 Shadow Boxing Exercises. They are credited to the Tang Dynasty (618-907 A.D.) and the Taoist Priest Xu Xuan Ping. For almost 1400 years, they have served as a reliable method of improving health and constitution, healing disease, and promoting longevity. This series when created was based on an even older Qigong set. The movements and imagery, which are inspired by nature, imitates the movements of the elephant, dragon, peacock, crane, horse, holding the moon, pushing a mountain, etc.

We practice with the purpose of making Qi flow smoothly through all the meridians. Although the standing postures are enough for the head massage practitioner, I would like to end this book by demonstrating some of our movements for the reader (See Figures 12-3 to 12-7).

There is a continuous and natural interplay between health, energy, and movement. This harmony is embodied in the Wu's Head Massage Sequence. Good health and good healing, it begins with a simple touch.

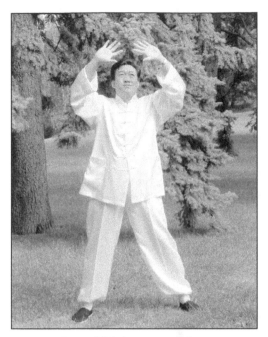

FIGURE 12-3 CIRCLING THE MOON

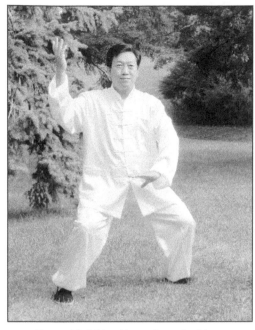

FIGURE 12-4 WILD HORSE PARTS ITS MANE

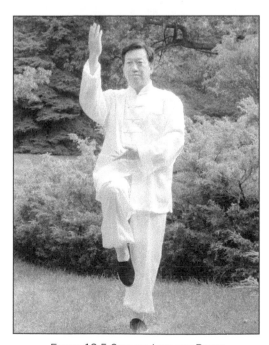

FIGURE 12-5 CIRCLING LEFT AND RIGHT

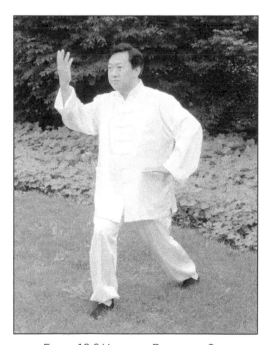

FIGURE 12-6 HOLDING A BALL AT THE SIDE

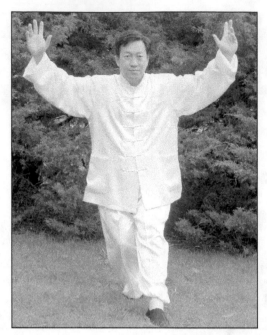

FIGURE 12-7 A ROC SPREADS ITS WINGS

References/Suggested Readings

The following books and articles have been used as reference guides in creating this book.

Historical Publications

Huang Di Nei Jing (*Yellow Emperor's Canon of Internal Medicine*)
Miraculous Pivot
Plain Questions
Highlights of Acupuncture
Compendium of Acupuncture and Moxibustion
Guide to the Classics of Acupuncture
Question and Answers Concerning Acupuncture and Moxibustion
Systematic Classics of Acupuncture

Contemporary Publications

Acupuncture and Moxibustion. First edition, edited by Nanjing College of Traditional Chinese Medicine, published by Shanghai Science and Technology Publishing House, 1974, Beijing

Acupoint Location Guide. Revised edition. Alon Lotan, 1995, published by Etsem.

Acupuncture and Moxibustion. First edition, edited by Shanghai College of Traditional Chinese Medicine, published by People's Medical Publishing House, 1974, Beijing.

Anatomical Charts for Acupuncture and Moxibustion. First edition, charted by Editorial and Charting Group of Anatomical Charts for Acupuncture and Moxibustion, Zhejiang Medical University, Zhejiang College of Traditional Chinese Medicine Publishing House, 1979, Hangzhou.

Anatomical Charts of Acupuncture of the 14 Meridians. Edited and charted by Shanghai College of Traditional Chinese Medicine, Shanghai Research Institute of Traditional Chinese Medicine, published by Shanghai People's Publishing House, 1975, Shanghai.

Chinese Acupuncture and Moxibustion. First edition, published by Foreign Languages Press, 1987, Beijing.

Essentials of Chinese Acupuncture. Published by People's Medical Publishing House, 1979, Beijing.

Explanation of Names of Acupoints with its English Translation. Published by Anhui Publishing House of Science & Technology, 1985, Anhui.

The English-Chinese Encyclopedia of Practical Traditional Chinese Medicine. First edition, published by Higher Education Press, 1994, Beijing.

A Practical English-Chinese Library of Traditional Chinese Medicine. First edition, published by Publishing House of Shanghai University of Traditional Chinese Medicine, 1990, Shanghai.

Additional Suggested Reading

(Not used as references for this book, but highly recommended reading)
Foundations of Traditional Chinese Medicine by Giovanni Maciocia
The Web That Has No Weaver by Ted Kaptchuk

Index

Author's Biographical Note

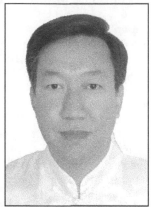

Dr. Bin Jiang Wu began his study of Traditional Chinese Medicine (TCM) and Qigong in his early childhood under the tutelage of TCM doctors within his family. He devoted numerous years to study under several renowned TCM doctors and Qigong Masters in China. His teachers include Professor Xue Tai Wang, Jin Zhang and the highly acclaimed TCM and Qigong Master, Guo Rui Jiao. He also learned from and befriended Xing Wan, a highly respected Shaolin Head Master. After a year as a "Barefoot Doctor" he began his formal education, and obtained his Doctor of Medicine from Heilongjiang University in 1983. In 1988, he graduated from the Masters Program in Medicine and Qigong from China Academy of TCM, Beijing. This was one of the first Masters Degrees of Medicine in Qigong offered in China and the world. In April 2000 after teaching and practicing TCM and Qigong in Europe and Japan, Dr. Wu became the President of the Ontario College of Traditional Chinese Medicine in Toronto, Canada. He uses his more than thirty years of experience in TCM to prepare Canadian and International students for a successful career and lifestyle based on the traditional healing principles of China.

Dr. Wu has dedicated many years to bridging the gap between the healing modalities of the East and West. He has held the position of Clinical Supervisor at Mount Sinai Hospital Pain Clinic and Michener Institute for Applied Health Sciences. He is currently the President of the Hungarian Qi Gong Association, Founder of the International Association of Acupuncture and Moxibustion Manipulative Techniques, Executive Director of the Chinese Medicine and Acupuncture Association of Canada, Executive Director of The Traditional Chinese Medicine Physicians Association of Canada, and an Honorary Professor of Acupuncture and Tuina at Heilongjiang University of TCM, China, and Founder and President of Wu's Head Massage International Association. He has also published over 20 papers on the effectiveness of TCM.

Dr. Wu's early experiences with the benefits of Tuina (Chinese Medicinal Massage) and with the treatment of "modern diseases" inspired him to develop Wu's Head Massage and to make it accessible to people worldwide.

"Teachers open the door ... You enter by yourself."

—*Chinese Proverb*

BOOKS FROM YMAA

more products available from...

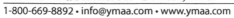

YMAA Publication Center, Inc. 楊氏東方文化出版中心

1-800-669-8892 • info@ymaa.com • www.ymaa.com

BOOKS FROM YMAA (continued)

DVDS FROM YMAA

more products available from…

YMAA Publication Center, Inc. 楊氏東方文化出版中心

1-800-669-8892 • info@ymaa.com • www.ymaa.com